Better Sex
Naturally

Chris D. Meletis, N.D.

Dean of Clinical Affairs,
Chief Medical Officer,
National College of Naturopathic
Medicine

with Susan M. Fitzgerald

Produced by The Philip Lief Group, Inc.

A Consumer's
Guide to
Herbs and
Other
Natural
Supplements that Can
Jump Start Your Sex Life

BETTER
Sex
Naturally

HarperResource
An Imprint of HarperCollins *Publishers*

This book is not intended to replace the services of a physician, nor is it meant to encourage diagnosis and treatment of illness, disease, or other medical problems. If you have any questions or concerns with any recommendation set forth in the following pages, and before taking any supplements, you should consult your physician. If you are under a physician's care for any condition, he or she can advise you whether the recommendations in this book are suitable for you.

BETTER SEX NATURALLY. © Copyright 2000 by The Philip Lief Group, Inc., and Chris Meletis, N.D. All rights reserved. Printed in the United States of America. No part of this book may be used or reproduced in any manner whatsoever without written permission except in the case of brief quotations embodied in critical articles and reviews. For information address HarperCollins*Publishers*, Inc., 10 East 53rd Street, New York, New York 10022.

HarperCollins books may be purchased for educational, business, or sales promotional use. For information, please write to: Special Markets Department, HarperCollins Publishers, Inc., 10 East 53rd Street, New York, New York 10022.

Produced by The Philip Lief Group, Inc.

Designed by Elina D. Nudelman

FIRST EDITION

Library of Congress Cataloging-in-Publication Data has been ordered.

ISBN 0–06–273688–4

00 01 02 03 04 ❖/RRD 10 9 8 7 6 5 4 3 2 1

*To my wife, Kathy, and
my sons, Nicholas and Matthew.
You are my inspiration.*

CONTENTS

ACKNOWLEDGMENTS

A special thanks to my wonderful and extremely patient wife, Kathy—your encouragement and friendship is priceless. I am grateful to my parents, Demetrios and Madeleine Meletis, for their loving guidance throughout my life.

This book could not have been completed without the assistance of many dedicated and talented people. I owe Susan Fitzgerald, a phenomenal writer, journalist, and friend, a huge thanks for all the talent, heart, and hard work that she imparted to this project, and for her amazing ability to breathe life into all the science and research supporting the wonders of natural medicine.

I would also like to acknowledge Scott Ferguson, N.D., for his assistance in gathering the research that substantiates the historical use of the herbs that have served humanity for centuries.

I am deeply appreciative of the tireless efforts and commitment of Judy Linden and Fiona Hinton of The Philip Lief Group, and the entire HarperCollins team.

I also give thanks to God for the blessings He has imparted and the bountiful resources provided for humanity's wellness in nature.

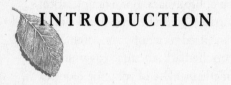

INTRODUCTION

Herbs Are Potent Medicine

You probably take echinacea to ward off a cold. Or St. John's Wort to beat the blues. Or Rescue Remedy® to keep your cool. It's only natural that you would look to herbal medicine to spice up your love life.

Natural healers around the world have long known there are many herbs that enhance sexual desire and performance in both men and women. For at least two thousand years, the Chinese used ginseng in their sex tonics to stimulate desire and build stamina. Since ancient times, natives of India have found ashwaganda a source of potency. More recently, in the Americas, Mexicans have used damiana to heighten their sexual experience, and in Brazil, muira puama has been known as "the herb of love."

The goal of *Better Sex Naturally* is to provide you with reliable information about long-revered aphrodisiacs that will not only improve your sex life but nourish your overall health, enhancing your entire sense of well-being. The knowledge of these successful remedies, gathered over countless generations by skilled herbal healers, is what scientists refer to as "empirical" knowledge. While empirical knowledge is not considered to be scientific, researchers appreciate it as fertile ground for study; the historical record of success can point them in the right direction. Scientific research is just beginning to document the effectiveness of herbal medicine, including aphrodisiacs. For example, local folklore that bark from Africa's yohimbe tree could stimulate erections in men inspired scientific research that resulted in a drug based on the bark, the first government-approved sex enhancing medicine. Use of yohimbe requires caution, as we will see in the chapter on this ancient aphrodisiac. It has since been supplanted by Pfizer Company's Viagra, whose use also requires caution in some individuals.

As we will find, herbs that work to enhance sexuality can also improve general health, and sometimes research into substances that improve health also finds that they can benefit sexual performance. For instance, researchers initially tested gingko leaf extract for its ability to increase memory through better circulation to the brain. But gingko's effect on circulation doesn't stop at the brain; it improves circulation all over the body, including the artery that delivers blood to the penis and clitoris, plus it strengthens the arteries that deliver the blood. When we are sexually aroused, blood rushes to the parts of the body that now have our complete attention, so for a pulse-pounding sexual experience, it makes sense to use herbs that not only increase blood flow but maximize the strength of the arterial delivery system.

In *Better Sex Naturally,* we will examine many herbs that have a track record for enhancing sexual desire and performance. To some, we have dedicated an entire chapter, including gingko biloba, ginseng, oat straw, and yohimbe. In other chapters, we have grouped herbs whose effects seem to be predominantly gender specific. In the "Especially for Men" chapter, we discuss saw palmetto, pygeum, muira puama, flower pollen, and stinging nettles. In "Especially for Women," we examine dong quai, wild yam, and black cohosh. In each chapter, we will:

1. Recount the historical use and folklore of the herb
2. Describe the chemistry and how it works in the body
3. Explain research that justifies the herb's aphrodisiac reputation
4. Identify side effects and possible negative interactions
5. Discuss tested dosages and available forms

As we examine each herb, we will frequently find that it acts over both the short and long term to improve sexual performance. This is because these herbs strengthen the body in ways specifically related to performance, and can also improve your overall health.

In a chapter called "Fact or Folklore," we will examine a few more substances that have some empirical evidence in their favor but await scientific validation. We will explore many of the same points as in the earlier chapters, such as historical use, chemistry, and safety. In the chapter called "Buyer Beware," we unlearn a few cultural myths; for example, Spanish fly does not live up to its reputation for inspiring uncontrollable sexual desire and can actually do harm.

Since sex is part of an overall healthy life, we will also hit some highlights about how you can keep your internal combustion engine running on all cylinders in the chapter called "To Your Health."

In Appendix A, "Putting It All Together—An Herbal Shopping List," I will run through my favorite herbs for women and men, as well as some of the popular combination herbal formulas on the market. In addition, I will list some guidelines for reading the labels on herbal products and other supplements.

As you may have read in both popular magazines and medical journals, there is great concern about herbal medicine in some quarters, ostensibly because herbal preparations do not provide standardized dosages of the active ingredients. Actually, there are many reliable manufacturers of herbal supplements who research, test, and standardize their products. As Dean of Clinical Affairs at the National College of Naturopathic Medicine, I can share with you which product lines we carry in our teaching clinics. This information can be found in Appendix B, "Resources for Further Information," which, as the title suggests, contains a host of other useful contacts, from naturopathic organizations to websites for natural medicine information.

Consult Appendix C for a glossary of terms used in *Better Sex Naturally*, and Appendix D for a bibliography of scientific papers and scientific and consumer texts used in the development of the book.

The Naturopathic Approach

My emphasis on overall health and how it affects sexual satisfaction stems from my training and philosophy as a naturopathic doctor (N.D.). Naturopathic doctors treat the whole person using gentle, natural substances to stimulate the body's own healing system. This concept of using the body's self-healing mechanisms is an ancient one, articulated in western culture as early as the fourth century B.C. by the Greek physician Hippocrates and later stated as the *vis medicatrix naturae*—the healing power of nature. Naturopathic physicians have embraced and honored this *vis medicatrix naturae* as the first principle from which the rest of our philosophy of medicine flows. Natural medicine offers so many benefits, and is in such demand, that many physicians who were not trained holistically are teaching themselves how to practice natural medicine. But natural medicine is more than substituting an herb for a pharmaceutically derived drug. The practice of naturopathic medicine is characterized by the following six principles, which are recurring themes as we explore how to use herbs to enhance sex.

1. The Healing Power of Nature.

   Central to the practice of naturopathic medicine is the belief that the human body has been created with the inherent ability to restore and maintain homeostatis, the optimal balance of all our systems. Homeostasis is the platform for optimal sex and optimal living, and herbal medicine has always played a vital role in supporting the *vis medicatrix naturae*.

2. Identify and Treat the Cause.

   Much of American medicine has been focused on symptoms and diseases, rather than causes. When it comes to sex, the most high-profile instance is the immediate and widespread popularity of Viagra. While this expensive, temporary remedy can have a place in the treatment of erectile dysfunction, it does not address the underlying cause of poor circulation in a long-term way. Left untreated, this cause can result in life-threatening conditions far more serious than a flaccid penis.

3. First, Do No Harm.

   It is the intention of the naturopathic physician to work with the body's own healing systems without disturbing other natural processes. Appropriately used, herbal means of enhancing the sexual experience do not upset any other physical system, unlike some of the mind-altering chemicals that people use, such as alcohol or cocaine.

4. Treat the Whole Person.

To function optimally, the human body in all its complexity must keep the mind, body, and spirit in balance. The herbs we recommend here have been shown historically and scientifically to have multi-faceted effects that promote overall health and sexual vitality.

5. The Physician as Teacher.

From the first moment of life onward, we are guests in bodies that somehow function miraculously each and every day. Since the human body doesn't come with an operating manual, it is the role of the physician, according to naturopathic philosophy, to educate patients how to restore and maintain optimal health. *Better Sex Naturally* is an extension of my role as a teacher to help you make choices that not only enhance your sexual experience but your entire well-being.

6. Prevention.

Building a strong foundation of health is fundamental to naturopathic medicine. The herbs recommended in this book can also strengthen your immune system, improve circulation, and arm you against stress-related diseases to help you maintain a long, healthy sex life.

These are ancient principles, and while naturopathic physicians make no exclusive claim to them, we are the only physicians whose training is imbued with them, who have formally adopted them, and practice according to them. The beneficiaries of this philosophy are our patients, whom we help motivate to make life-changing choices for health.

The Education of a
Naturopathic Doctor

A naturopathic doctor's scientific training is comparable to that of medical doctors and osteopathic doctors. We all study a similar amount of graduate-level anatomy, physiology, pathology, biochemistry, pharmacology, and diagnostics. Naturopathic doctors are the only licensed primary care physicians who are additionally trained in holistic methods to address the causes of "dis-ease" and to promote health. These gentle, natural treatment methods flow from the principles to honor the healing power of nature and to do no harm:

1. Botanical medicine

2. Clinical nutrition

3. Physical medicine (such as therapeutic manipulation of muscle, bone and tissues, heat and cold, microcurrent, ultrasound, and traction)

4. Mind-body medicine (counseling, stress management, biofeedback)

5. Homeopathy

In addition to these treatment methods, we also are trained to use standard laboratory and diagnostic tests, and in Oregon, where I am licensed, to prescribe many standard pharmaceuticals, such as antibiotics, hormones, and pain medications.

So what's all this philosophy got to do with *Better Sex Naturally?* It's simple: The better we feel, the greater will be our sexual satisfaction. The goal of naturopathic medicine is to help people to reach their optimal level of health, which prepares them to experience life more fully, including sex.

In Chapter One, "The Right Chemistry," we will examine the workings of the body's sexual system, how herbs can affect it, and how we can go from good sex to better sex, maybe even the best!

1 THE RIGHT CHEMISTRY

It's Saturday morning, and you and your partner are getting the chores done when she distracts you by bending over to pick up your socks—there's just something about that position that gives you a tingle. She swings her head back up and you see the bounce in her hair, the curve of her hip, and as she walks by, you impulsively reach out to her. She pauses and smiles, so you take the opportunity for a hug. Unconsciously, or maybe not, you pick up each other's scent, and as she moves into you, you get the idea she'd like more than a hug. A warm, full-bodied kiss cranks both your engines and the next thing you know, you are messing up the freshly made bed.

Any combination of things could happen next, but what we're going to talk about is the chemistry required to get us to this point. For both men and women, the sex drive is fueled by testosterone, so he feels that tingle and she responds to that hug, but sexual responsiveness takes more than testosterone. Healthy adrenal glands release the chemicals that trigger the special scent that some researchers believe we each have. Mental alertness to sexual cues and responses is required, so that when she bends over, he notices, and when she pulls him closer, he knows what that means. Both partners feel relaxed and comfortable with each other and who they are. They have the physical energy to pursue what their chemistry has set in motion, and the healthy heart and arteries to pump the blood and deliver the hormonal messages to where they need to go.

If our most basic instinct is this complicated, it simply underscores the importance of keeping all the equipment operating at peak efficiency. Herbs can be a vital ingredient in the mix. Let's look at each ingredient in this chemical cocktail and get a glimpse of what herbs can bring to the party.

Testosterone

Testosterone is the key ingredient in men's and women's sex drive. In men, it also acts as an anti-depressant, making them feel optimistic. While much is written of women's hormonal fluctuations, men have no room to point fingers—testosterone levels can fluctuate greatly throughout any given day. Abnormally low levels of testosterone will have a marked effect on men's outlook and sex drive, depressing both their mood and their libido.

We know that women's sex drive stems largely from testosterone, because even if the ovaries, which produce estrogen, are removed, a woman's sex drive can be unimpaired. But take the testosterone-producing adrenal glands out of the picture, and she can kiss her sex drive goodbye! Estrogen does play a role in sexual health, however; low levels can cause diminished lubrication and vaginal atrophy, in which the vaginal walls become thinner; this means that friction will cause injury, pain, and possible bleeding.

One way to keep testosterone activity up is to take ginseng. The ancient Chinese used ginseng as a sexual tonic.

This herb is so potent that in laboratory experiments, even castrated rats go into a mating frenzy. While ginseng hasn't been shown to be hormone-like, it is known to accentuate testosterone activity, which increases the effectiveness with which the body releases and uses the hormone.

Adrenal Glands

The adrenal glands are small, almond-sized organs that have a big impact on our system. They are located directly above (*ad*) the kidneys (*renal*), hence their name. The adrenals produce a variety of hormones—we have many more of them than just the gender-oriented testosterone and estrogen—that regulate many physical responses. One non-gender hormone that most people know about is adrenaline and the "fight or flight" response that triggers its release. Adrenaline has an indirect impact on sexual preparedness. For example, if that "fight or flight" response gets triggered on the way home from work by some road rage, the adrenaline rush causes the arteries to constrict, keeping blood from the extremities so it is available for the brain and internal organs. This works well as a protective mechanism, but it certainly doesn't do much for the "extremities" if your partner wants to hit the hay as soon as you hit the door! Even hours after that enraging traffic, after you think you've calmed down, your body is still reeling from the hormones that flooded your system.

"Tonic" herbs such as India's ashwagandha can come to the rescue. The tonic effect is described as balancing the system, relaxing it if it is stressed, and energizing it if it is fatigued, both of which result from an adrenaline rush. If your stressful life results in frequent adrenaline hits, it is also a good idea to include plenty of nutrients such as Vitamin C and pantothenic acid from fresh fruits, vegetables, and nuts to preserve adrenal health.

The adrenal glands also produce dehydroepiandrosterone (DHEA), which has received a lot of publicity as the "anti-aging" hormone. It is a basic ingredient of other sex-related hormones such as progesterone. As a building block, some scientists believe there is more DHEA in our bodies than any other hormone. Sufficient DHEA levels have been implicated in pheromone production, the "sexy smell" chemical that some researchers theorize makes people feel attracted to each other. Some scientists think humans no longer have this capability and that only animals emit pheromones as a method of attracting each other for sex. Others continue research to document that human pheromones still exist. Marketers aren't waiting around for human proof. They're convinced by lab research that shows pheromones are so powerful that insects can detect them even miles away, and they are banking on humans to buy pheromone-based colognes.

Be Alert!

The brain is the body's biggest sex organ. It's true—the limbic system of the brain rules desire and emotion. Women know this but some men still scoff. Let me pose this question, gentlemen: If Pamela Anderson or Sandra Bullock walked into your room and gave you a scorching "come-hither" stare, would you get that tingle if your brain didn't give the high sign? Nope. It's the brain that triggers the release of testosterone, kicking off the chemical reaction that results in that tingle and the urge to do something about it.

This communication system can be affected by many of the chemicals we use all the time. Just think of the combination of legal drugs we might ingest in the course of a day— the coffee, the colas, the tobacco (first- or secondhand), the allergy/sinus/cold medications. They can take a toll:

1. Nicotine constricts the blood vessels.
2. Caffeine can promote anxiety.
3. Antihistamines can put you to sleep or make you buzz like a bee.

Sometimes we take drugs such as alcohol, marijuana, or cocaine with the hope of enhancing our sexual satisfaction. While these can relax our inhibitions, they also numb our senses, so even if we're uninhibited enough to have great sex, how will we know? And, as many lovers have found to their sorrow, these substances don't list the "medicinal" dose at which inhibitions are down and capability is still up. For a really mind-blowing sexual experience, kick these brain-foggers and try gingko.

Gingko has become widely renowned in the past few decades for its ability to promote mental alertness. It does this by relaxing the arteries to improve blood flow to the brain, in addition to actually stimulating blood flow. Of course, this has implications beyond the cerebral cortex; gingko also improves blood flow to the genitals of both men and women. Women joke that men think with their crotch instead of their brains because blood can't flow in two places at once. Gingko may be the answer to this problem! Gingko does more than promote blood flow; it makes you more alert, more interested, more vibrant, and ready for whatever comes up.

Relax!

Stress can be death to your sex drive. That is because the body's responses to stress increases adrenaline production and diminish blood flow to parts the body considers unnecessary in a crisis, which, of course, includes the genitals. Chronic stress causes stubborn physical problems:

1. Wildly fluctuating hormone levels are too unbalanced to easily restore, so you always feel tired, and your ability to deal with continual stress diminishes.

2. Blood vessels remain constricted and do not "bounce back" to pre-stress capacity as readily, posing a barrier to healthy circulation for all your organs.

3. Both hormone levels and vasoconstriction affect the body's means of stimulating arousal and erection in both sexes, and lubrication in women.

4. Tempers grow short, emotions fluctuate, fatigue sets in—all of which can kill not only the mood, but you, too, if left untreated.

Aside from the physical effects of everyday stress, good sex also results from two people being relaxed and comfortable, not only with who they are but how they feel when they're together. You care about each other and want to make each other feel good. This works for people young and old, fit or fat, rich or poor, bald or bushy. Nobody's watching the clock to see how long you can do it, in how many positions, or who falls asleep first.

One herb we discuss that has a soothing effect on the body and mind is oat straw, or what used to be called "wild oats." *Avena sativa*, to give oats their botanical name, is the basis of oatmeal. Use of the whole plant had medicinal qualities, such as a mild sedative effect, and nutrients that support nervous system functions. If you're feeling the effects of stress, you may want to sow wild oats!

Rest!

Sleep helps you fight the effects of stress and fatigue. It improves your mood, raises your sexual energy, and increases mental and physical energy. While there is no substitute for a good night's sleep, there are herbs that promote energy, such as gotu kola. Gotu kola has antioxidant and anti-inflammatory properties and is used in both Ayurvedic and Chinese medicine as an energizing sexual tonic.

Hearts and Arteries

Circulation, circulation, circulation! Without it, the blood doesn't effectively make the rounds of the miles of vessels in our body that bring nutrients, carry away waste, and nourish the heart, kidneys, liver, and lungs. Circulatory health is like the oil in your car's engine—if your system gets sluggish and the arteries clog up, functions all over your body start to slow down or go haywire. It's gradual, and sometimes the changes are chalked up to age, but it's really an issue of lifestyle choices; circulation responds readily to changes in diet and exercise. Sometimes it doesn't get any attention until the one thing a man counts on, that reliable erection, starts to flag. Women may wonder where their sex drive went; they still have the urge, but not the energy, to merge. Even before that point, however, you may experience some loss of stamina. To keep those pipes clear, gingko may be the prescription for you.

As you can see, gingko is the key to a basic function, circulation (and it's one of the oldest documented sex tonic ingredients), so that is where we will start our search for *Better Sex Naturally*.

2 GINGKO BILOBA

Hug this tree!
Gingko can improve
your sex life,
your memory,
and help fight cancer!

Gingko biloba is a great example of a "tonic" herb—one that balances whatever is going on in your system; if you're tired, it can energize you; if you're stressed, it can relax you. It is an overall "good for what ails you" herb with not only 2,000 years of empirical observation, but with more than 400 studies to validate its reputation, some of which uphold its use as a sex tonic.

Gingko's hallmark effect is increased circulation, which can be a tremendous boost to optimal health because blood is the vehicle that carries nourishment to every cell in our body, and our circulatory system is the delivery route to those cells. With our busy lives these days, we need all the help we can get to maintain our energy level. The better our circulation, the more we benefit from the good food we choose to eat and the vitamins and herbal supplements we take—and the better we are prepared for the heart-racing excitement of sex.

For men, especially, circulation's effect on sex is "make or break." If the arteries start getting clogged, erections can become iffy. Gingko helps relax and dilate arterial walls to get the blood flowing. And it's not only men who benefit: Women using gingko report an increase in multiple orgasms, according to Robyn Landis in *Herbal Defense*. She reports that anecdotal evidence points to increased intensity and duration of orgasm in both men and women.

A Living Fossil

Gingko biloba (bi-loba=two-lobed leaf) is the last remaining species of the Ginkoales order, a deciduous conifer that is at least 200 million years old. Fossil records show the species was widespread in Asia and North America. It was thought to be extinct, and it is speculated that monks in far eastern temples cultivated it secretly as a sacred tree.

Gingko biloba is an odd-looking conifer. It can be as much as 10–12 stories high, yet its trunk is only three to four feet in diameter and its branches are relatively short. Its creamy white flowers bloom at night; its fruit is yellow, inedible, and smells horrible, but the kernel is used as both food and medicine.

It is difficult to cultivate gingko commercially; it lives for hundreds of years, so it can take decades before there is something to harvest. Commercial gingko has usually been wildcrafted, that is, harvested in its natural habitat, in Asia, Europe, and North America.

Ancient Roots

The earliest known reference to gingko's medicinal use is the 2,800 B.C. Chinese Materia Medica, which is a sort of herbal encyclopedia of medicinal plants and their uses and preparations. In addition to the medicinal use of the root, the Chinese, Japanese, and Koreans all savored the kernel of the fruit, raw or cooked, as an everyday food. Ancient Asians roasted the kernel and ate it to aid digestion and prevent drunkenness. The Chinese believed the kernel nourished sexual vitality. A decoction of the root—a kind of tea—was used to support the kidney function of filtering impurities out of the body. The Chinese also saw a spiritual aspect in the bi-lobed leaf, representing "two becoming one," a fitting analogy for a plant believed to increase sexual energy.

The tree was introduced into Europe in 1730 as an ornamental specimen, and today we see it lining city streets all over North America, favored for its resiliency against pollutants and pests.

Chinese medicinal use of the root and seed is ancient, although use of the leaf is scarcely 20 years old. A concentrated extract of gingko leaf has been studied widely in recent years for its cardiovascular benefits, and is prescribed on a daily basis by thousands of doctors worldwide.

Today, gingko is among the top five most commonly prescribed herbal medicines in Germany and France. German physicians prescribe gingko over 5 million times a year, while U.S. physicians scarcely recommend it at all.

How It Works

Gingko leaf extract has received much attention as a result of research that documents its ability to improve memory. It does this by dilating cerebral blood vessels, which increases blood flow to the brain. The active ingredients of gingko are flavone glycosides, bioflavones, sitosterol, lactones, and anthocyanins. Gingko also contains more of a circulation-enhancing chemical called terpene lactone than other plants. Interestingly, the scientific evidence that documents ginkgo's effect on relaxing cerebral arterial walls and improving circulation to the brain also led researchers to the knowledge that gingko improves the circulation to peripheral tissues necessary to supply blood to men's and women's sex organs.

Several studies demonstrate the power of gingko leaf extract to help men who have circulation problems affecting their ability to get erections. The men in these studies took gingko for a specified period of time to get these results, but as the research also shows, the herb starts going to work within an hour to improve circulation. This bodes well for men and women who already have good sex and seek to enhance their experience. Here are the most often cited research results:

- One German study reported that in a six-month period, 50 percent of men regained their ability to achieve erections while on gingko extract. Another 25 percent, who were not responding to injections of another chemical, papaverine, into the base of the penis to dilate the artery, were able to get erections using the shots and gingko in combination.

James Duke, Ph.D., author of *The Green Pharmacy*, recounts other pertinent research:

- In one nine-month study, 78 percent of men significantly improved their ability to get erections without adverse effects.

- One study demonstrated that blood flow through the capillaries increased by 57 percent only one hour after administration of gingko to healthy adults.

If gingko can help these men, think what it can do for you! From this research, we also can extrapolate gingko's benefits to women, in whom the herb's circulatory effects can increase lubrication and clitoral stimulation and heighten orgasm. While gingko starts going to work quickly, this is an herb that provides its maximum benefits when taken over a period of at least six months. And while you're improving your sex life, you will also be enjoying overall increased vitality and mental alertness.

That was the experience of Jack, a 52-year-old who thought he was too young to be as forgetful and lethargic as he was. His work was suffering, and he was having a hard time keeping up in the softball league he had played in for years. As we talked about what was going on in his life, which is typical when visiting a naturopathic doctor, Jack casually mentioned he was feeling some disappointment in his sexual energy, too. All he could say was that "it" didn't work very well. Neither of us was content to write "it" off as yet another example of the 31 percent or so of men over 50 who "don't work very well."

I prescribed a standardized 24% gingko extract of 60 mg four times a day, and sent him off with the assignment of drinking more water, decreasing stress, and taking that gingko faithfully. When Jack returned a month later for his follow-up visit, I could tell right away he was a much happier man. Sure enough, he not only reported improved memory and energy, but was beginning to experience the sexual benefits of the herb, too.

Gingko has some other interesting effects, according to Daniel Reid's *Handbook of Chinese Healing Herbs*:

1. Enhanced sperm production, as a result of antioxidant action and nutrients provided by the herb.

2. Help in controlling nocturnal emissions by modulating tissue sensitivity and improving muscle tone.

3. Improvement in cases of involuntary or premature ejaculation. This is probably the result of improved mental clarity and focus, helping to break what some researchers call a "bad habit" developed in adolescence in response to less-than-optimal conditions for sex (i.e., worry that parents might come home early, or the partner might change their mind).

Research: Sexy Results

Scientists started studying gingko because of the circulatory benefits to cardiac and stroke patients. But, after more than 400 studies, its benefits to sexual performance have not escaped notice. Various gingko preparations have been tested and found to:

1. Significantly increase creation and production of dopamine, adrenaline, and other neurotransmitters in the brain, which are often associated with pleasure, arousal, and increased alertness.

2. Increase blood flow in the capillary vessels and end-arteries, accounting for its demonstrable effect on the venous system, which is involved with achieving erection.

3. Help regulate the tone and elasticity of the blood vessels, making them work more efficiently.

4. Act as an antidote to some of the effects of alcohol intoxication (which has been known to dampen not a few sexual episodes!), as a result of gingko's antioxidant properties, which can lessen the toxic accumulation of aldehydes, the substances created by the breakdown of alcohol that lead to hangovers.

Fine-Tuning Health

We think of health as simply being the absence of symptoms, but to a naturopathic doctor, that's just the baseline in determining optimal wellbeing. Take Julie, for example. At 23, she was beginning her career as a computer animation artist. She took vitamins and jogged regularly, so she wondered why she didn't have more energy. "I just felt kind of tired a lot and overwhelmed," she said. "I wanted to be in a relationship, but it seemed like work was all I could handle. I didn't feel sick, but I didn't feel especially well, either." In talking about her desire for a steady relationship, Julie said her past sexual experiences were rewarding but felt she hadn't yet peaked in that area.

Clearly, Julie was motivated to achieve optimal health, and her efforts just needed a little fine-tuning. As we examined her health profile, we determined that the birth control pills she took to keep her periods regular probably drained her of more B-complex vitamins than she was taking in from food or supplements. The connection between B vitamins and stress is well-documented: if you are stressed, you deplete yourself of B vitamins, and if you are low in B, you have a harder time fighting stress. Those vanilla lattes Julie loved didn't help. Caffeine drains B vitamins and its diuretic effect can result in slight, ongoing dehydration that will make a person feel fatigued. Caffeine also constricts the blood vessels, so nutrients and oxygen weren't adequately circulated.

Together, Julie and I worked out a plan she could live with: increase her B-complex intake, cut down to a single latte a day followed by lots of water, and add gingko supplements to offset the chronic blood vessel constriction caused by the caffeine and to boost her energy levels. I suspected that Julie would be taking the gingko long enough before her next relationship that she would be experiencing some sexual benefits as well. She confirmed that suspicion on a follow-up visit some months later. "It was very gradual," she said. "One day after a few weeks, I just found myself bouncing out of bed." When she met a man who eventually became her partner, she found the sex was more physically exciting and rewarding. "Everything just felt better, more alive," she said.

Side Effects

The doses of standardized Gingko Biloba Extract (GBE) used in studies to achieve clinical effects mentioned in this chapter are often large, and still researchers have reported no serious side effects. A few very rare and minor discomforts have been noted in the research literature:

1. Mild gastrointestinal upset in less than 1% of patients in clinical studies.

2. Slight headaches for patients with poor blood flow to the brain for first 1–2 days of use.

3. Diarrhea, irritability, and restlessness may be caused by large amounts (above 240 mg per day) of standardized extract.

Not for Everyone

There are some contraindications and negative interactions you should be aware of before you rush off to the health food store for a lifetime supply of gingko.

Aspirin

Chronic use of aspirin with gingko may lead to an increased chance of bleeding. Aspirin prevents platelets from sticking together, and so does gingko. There could be a cumulative effect if both are taken regularly, and a handful of such cases have been reported.

Monoamine Oxidase Inhibitors

MAO inhibitors are an entire family of anti-depressants used for treatment of depression and panic disorders. They are also used to treat vascular or tension headaches. Some researchers speculate that because gingko improves circulation to the brain, patients who are using MAO inhibitors may have increased amounts of the drug delivered to the brain, leading to toxicity from an otherwise safe dose.

Medical Conditions

There are a few medical conditions for which gingko may be inadvisable:

Stroke.

Gingko use should be monitored in high-risk stroke patients, because they may be taking blood thinners such as warfarin, and the synergistic effect with gingko may further thin the blood.

Hemorrhage.

As previously mentioned, gingko thins the blood, so it could be contraindicated for a person who has a tendency to hemorrhage.

The Formula That Works

Gingko biloba leaf must be taken in a more concentrated form than is found in nature to get the vasodilatory effect. This is probably why it was not used in ancient Chinese medicine. Leaves (fresh or dried), harvested in summer, are often made into standardized tincture, or fluid extract. It takes about 50 pounds of gingko leaves to create one pound of standardized GBE (Gingko biloba extract). Reducing the leaves to a usable formula requires a 27-step extraction process that may take up to two weeks. Fortunately, you can find GBE in your local health food store or grocery store in capsules of 40 mg to 120 mg.

When you are comparing product prices, be sure to look for a formula with 24% flavonglycosides. Flavonglycosides are the chemicals that give the leaf its color and tangy taste, and which researchers identify as the active ingredient, and at 24% these will produce the documented effects. The most frequent dose used in studies and in the clinical setting is 40 mg, 3 times a day, of the standardized extract, and GBE has been found safe to be used at that level for as long as medically indicated. In clinical tests, men with circulation-related erection problems took as little as 60 mg per day. The dose indicated for your unique needs will vary depending on your overall health.

Standardized Forms (capsules):
    Gingko 24% (standardized), 40–60 mg, 3–4 times a day

Tincture (50:1) Concentrate:
    Alcohol or Glycerite Extract, 30 drops, 3–4 times a day

Tincture (2:1) Regular Extract:
    60–90 drops, 4 times a day

Gingko Tea:
    1 tbs of leaf, steeped, 3–4 times a day

Gingko (dried, nonstandardized herb):
    1000 mg, 1–2 times a day

Is Gingko Right for Me?

We examine many herbs in this book and the question naturally arises, "Which one should I take?" First, it is wise to consult with your physician before taking any substance you expect to have a medicinal effect. My approach is to examine the patient's entire health profile; if I see an occasional occurrence, or family history, of the following conditions, I believe this indicates a higher probability the patient will benefit from gingko's circulatory benefits:

- Short-term memory loss
- Vertigo
- Headache
- Ringing in the ears (tinnitus)
- Depression
- Varicose veins
- Cold hands or feet

In keeping with the naturopathic principle of prevention, taking gingko can help keep these conditions at bay, while enhancing sexual health.

3 GINSENG

I would rather take
a handful of ginseng
than a cartload
of gold and jewels.

—*OLD CHINESE PROVERB*—

Ginseng is reputed to have boosted the potency of Ottoman sultans, the stamina of Olympic athletes, and the GPA of Chinese students. More than 1,000 studies in the past 30 years validate ginseng's 5,000-year-old reputation among the ancient Chinese as the king of herbs, a "sovereign" remedy for almost any ill. Ginseng's botanical name, *panax*, indicates its broad therapeutic value: The word *panax* comes from the same word as the Greek goddess Panacea, healer of all.

Ginseng, in its several varieties, is classified as an adaptogenic herb, one that increases the body's ability to adapt to environmental stresses and correct biochemical imbalances. It energizes when you are fatigued and calms when you are over-anxious. Adaptogens are nontoxic substances that reinforce the body's ability to adapt to any stressor. Ginseng also increases the production of sex-related hormones like testosterone and enhances sexual response in both men and women. Ginseng is one of the most important tonic herbs used in Chinese sexual therapy and aphrodisiacs, according to master Chinese herbalist Ron Teeguarden in *Radiant Health*.

Fit for a Sultan

An aphrodisiac still peddled in the streets of Istanbul uses ginseng as an important ingredient. Those who sell the "Royal Love Potion" allege its formula was concocted by the imperial doctor to help a sultan maintain a majestic virility with his harem.

Ancient Roots

Chinese lore relates that ginseng was so prized that only emperors had the right to collect the roots of this esteemed herb. The Chinese called ginseng "man root" because they thought the root system looked like a human body. Native American tribes must have thought so, too; they gave the North American species of the plant an equivalent name. Ginseng's root is the medicinal part of this perennial herb. It was chewed by the sick to recover health and by the healthy to increase their vitality, says M. Grieve in *A Modern Herbal*. Chinese university students chew on the root while studying for exams because they say it heightens their concentration and memory.

Ginseng is native to China, Siberia, Manchuria, and North America. The Asian species is larger than the American species, but they are both similar in appearance: a large, fleshy root that can grow to be several inches thick, topped by a simple stem about a foot high, bearing three leaves divided into fine-toothed leaflets, and red berries. Ginseng is slow to mature and the biggest roots make the best medicine. The Chinese herbal practitioners refuse to use roots less than seven years old, believing that the more mature roots are more potent. The root's bitter taste is offset by a sweet, licorice-like flavor. Ginseng grows best in hilly woodlands, and in North America it can be found on mountain slopes from Quebec to Georgia.

There are a variety of species, and those most commonly used in herbal preparations are *Panax* (Chinese), *Eleuthrococcus* (Siberian), and *Panax quinquafolium* (North American). Wild *panax* is the rarest, and most prized, variety. It can grow to 65 years old and will fetch thousands of dollars for less than an ounce of root in markets where it is prized, such as Hong Kong. Although ginseng requires demanding soil and climate conditions, farmers in the United States, Canada, Japan, and Korea are cultivating it with some success. The U.S. exports more than $100 million worth of its native wild *panax quinquafolius* to Asian markets every year. In 1996, 1,400 farmers in Wisconsin alone grew 1.6 million pounds of ginseng, valued at $90 million; 87 percent of it was exported to Asia. Ginseng is sold in products such as powders, tonics, tablets, teas, liquid extracts, and even fruit drinks and confections, plus the plain root, generating world-wide sales of $3.75 billion, according to *The Economist*.

A Constant Adventure

The power of ginseng is the stuff of legend in Asia. Chinese soldiers took ginseng into battle with them, and Russian cosmonauts took it into space. At the turn of the century, three Cossacks were murdered in Siberia for selling an inferior root. A story in the November 21, 1998 issue of the British medical journal <u>Lancet</u> recounts one man's acquisition of a 20-inch-long ginseng root from Indonesia. It was so old that the root system was squid-like, and the cost of the root was the equivalent of two years' pay for the locals. The locals' reverence for the root was evidenced in its packaging: a box lined with red velvet. According to Chinese folklore, such a grand root could be cut only by a silver knife.

How It Works

Researchers have identified as many as 20 varieties of a chemical component called triterpenoid saponins, which are abundant in all types of ginseng and which are the "active ingredients" believed responsible for the herb's adaptogenic qualities. Like many of the herbs we examine, ginseng has multiple effects: It acts as a tonic (system balancer), a stimulant, and an aphrodisiac. It stimulates secretions from the salivary glands and gallbladder, which improve digestion and elimination of body wastes. It enhances the immune response by stimulating components such as natural killer cells—T cells and phagocytes—which help fight off viruses and bacteria. Like gingko, it relaxes the arteries to improve blood pressure and circulation.

Ginseng has a marked effect on several metabolic functions, including our stress response, which accounts for its reputation as an energizing herb:

Adrenal glands.

As we discussed in Chapter One, maintaining healthy adrenal health is crucial to maintaining and enhancing our sexual vitality. Ginseng supports the adrenal gland function to lessen excess adrenaline release; adrenaline hikes blood pressure and modulates blood sugar, resulting in feelings of fatigue.

Stamina.

Ginseng enhances the body's use of glycogen, a carbohydrate we use as a fuel reserve. Glycogen is stored in the liver and muscles until our energy demands, during sex for example, require that glycogen be transformed into glucose to fuel our activity. Ginseng helps by increasing the amount of glycogen in the liver by 83 percent and in the muscles by 33 percent in controlled studies, making more energy available to us.

Energy.

Ginseng works in two ways to increase available energy: (1) by improving oxygen use throughout the body, which improves mental clarity and enhanced physical endurance for strenuous activity; and (2) by decreasing the inhibitory effect of low-density lipoproteins (a cholesterol) released when we are stressed, which hinder the body's ability to release energy stored in cells.

As science uncovers links between body chemistry and emotions like anxiety, we find that ginseng's reputation as a "nerve tonic" is also justified. Clinical observations of patients with various nervous or psychic disorders benefited from the balancing effects of ginseng. These individuals were characterized by unbalanced moods, anxiety, and irritability. They tended to tire easily, and many had problems with insomnia. After a course of treatment with ginseng, signs of depression and sluggishness were eliminated or significantly relieved, and the herb produced a sedating effect with emotionally excited patients.

Different Philosophies

Over and over again, you will see that the herbs we examine in this book have many medicinal effects. To a holistic healer, this is one of the wonders of nature. Chinese medical practitioners view an herb like ginseng as a superior remedy—one that supports the body's effort to fight whatever comes. An inferior remedy would be one that addresses only one specific condition. Ironically, this is what too many doctors and researchers value most—the magic bullet. They think if an herb is good for everything, it can't be good for anything. So they try to isolate the "magic bullet" part of an herb to test it, but sometimes they find out that just one chemical element of an herb is not as effective as the entire root, leaf, or flower, so they write off the oldest branch of medicine as worthless. Someday, maybe that view will be considered as ridiculous as bleeding people with leeches to cure them.

Even Varro Tyler, Ph.D., Sc.D., "America's foremost expert on herbs," is "convinced ginseng may have some value as a tonic," as he said in *Prevention,* August 1997. He recounted several reliable studies in the 1990s that show ginseng, in combination with vitamins and minerals, improved research subjects' quality of life in the areas of fatigue reduction, improved memory, and general psychological sense of wellbeing.

Research: Sexy Results

In Soviet studies of Siberian ginseng (*Eleutherococcus)* use by hundreds of athletes, including Olympic contenders, research confirmed ginseng's reputation as an energizer that increases endurance, hones reflexes, and improves concentration. Athletes noted that they were able to increase the amount and duration of training while using ginseng. These athletes were at the pinnacle of what most of us would consider optimal health, and still ginseng improved their stamina and reflexes. If you want to perform Olympic feats in your own arena, ginseng is a strong contender as your herb of choice.

Chinese experiments using ginseng in humans have shown:

- Increased production of a luteinizing hormone produced by the pituitary gland in the brain, which stimulates progesterone in women.

- Increased testosterone secretion in men and women.

- Improved muscle development.

Ginseng also acts to increase fertility and productivity, as shown in animal studies in which:

- Cows produced more milk.
- Bees produced more honey.
- Bulls produced more semen, up to 28 percent.
- Mice gre w heavier testicles.

SAD story

Carla and Mike had a rollicking sex life, making love several times a week—as long as the sun shone. "Just like clockwork, Carla's sex drive goes into hibernation around Thanksgiving and didn't come back until Easter," Mike complained. "I don't know why I'm like this," Carla said. "Mike thinks it's hormones and I should get fixed." It sounded like a SAD case to me. Seasonal Affective Disorder, prevalent in northern climates, offers simple, reproducible proof that your mind controls your sex life. Several times from October to February, I see patients suffering this downward spiral.

SAD is caused by lack of exposure to full spectrum natural light. As the days darken and nights lengthen, some people experience decreased production of the hormone melatonin, secreted by a part of the brain called the pineal gland. SAD is also associated with an increased secretion of cortisol by the adrenal glands, which disturbs the blood sugar level and can result in a feeling of fatigue, weakness, and lethargy.

We combined a couple of therapeutic methods to shift Carla from SAD to glad. A light box, which introduced full-spectrum lighting to mimic the natural sunlight that Carla craved, helped reset her natural rhythms. I also prescribed melatonin to offset the seasonal deficiency of this hormone, and ginseng to support the function of the adrenal glands, thereby reducing the secretion of cortisol. It took only a few weeks for this treatment to light up Mike and Carla's love life all year round.

Side Effects

Ginseng is exceptionally safe, and side effects are very rare. Though almost all ginseng varieties are non-toxic, Siberian ginseng appears to be the least problematic. In fact, a healthy adult would have to eat about four-and-one-half pounds of ginseng at a sitting, or about twelve pounds in the case of Siberian ginseng, to reach a lethal dosage.

Occasionally, there can be sensations of slight drowsiness immediately after taking a dose. You can offset this effect by taking the herb with meals if you find this to be your experience.

Not for Everyone

Chinese herbalists recommend that ginseng not be used by those who get spontaneous nose bleeds, and women with excessive menstrual bleeding, except under the guidance of a professional. Ginseng would not be recommended for anyone diagnosed with high blood pressure, extra heartbeats, rapid heart rate, or muscle tension. If sleep problems are an issue, do not use ginseng within four hours of bedtime. Also, a small study showed that one out of six people who consume caffeine with 3 grams of ginseng dried herb over a period of weeks will develop increased blood pressure.

Possible drug interactions can occur for those taking medication for these diseases:

Diabetes.
Since ginseng can lower blood sugar, it may be necessary to work with your physician to adjust your insulin levels.

Manic Depression.
If used with an MAO inhibitor, ginseng may increase the likelihood of manic symptoms.

Heart disease.

Blood thinners such as Warfarin, also known as coumadin, may have their effects reduced by ginseng, and caution is advised.

The Formula That Works

When you start looking for ginseng, you will find a wide variety of formulas. There are some differences of opinion on which species of ginseng produce which effects (See "To Each His Own Ginseng"). Some clinicians say that if a person tends to be chilly, then *panax* is a better choice than Siberian ginseng. If you find a ginseng formula with the following ingredients in the proper ratios, you should be able to enjoy the benefits of this herb.

A typical dose should contain at least 10 mg of ginenoside Rg1, with a 1:2 ratio of Rg1: Rb1. You can take this dose one to three times a day. This balance can be found in the following (concentrated) forms:

Tinctures:
Alcohol Herbal Extracts; 30–60 drops a day, depending on concentration.

Syrups:
Sweet liquid solutions concentrated for potency; strengths vary greatly; follow directions on the label or ask your practitioner.

Capsules:
Standardized capsules of concentrated powder; 10–50 milligrams; 1–3 times a day.

Dried herb (not concentrated):
500–1000 milligrams in capsule or tea form; 1–2 times a day.

All these formulas will increase energy, sense of wellbeing, and sexual invigoration.

Although some people experience immediate results, it is best to continue use for one week to one month. Ginseng's effects will continue for a time even after you have stopped taking it. A regimen of two to three month periods of use followed by a month without the product is ideal. This is because ginseng is basically restorative in nature and slowly helps to build greater health.

As ginseng's energizing qualities became widely known, manufacturers started putting it in products ranging from soft drinks to candy bars and selling them as "natural" energy foods. But ginseng isn't the only "natural" ingredient; check the labels for caffeine, sugar, chocolate, and other stimulants. You might consider taking your ginseng "straight up" without any added ingredients.

To Each His Own Ginseng

Some herbalists say that ginseng varieties act specifically on certain physical functions and that we should take this into account when we are assessing what effect we want to achieve. Stephen Fulder, in his 1996 The Ginseng Book, explains that American ginseng (*panax quinquefolius*) is considered more "yin" or cooling and rejuvenating, and Asian ginseng (*panax ginseng*) is considered more "yang" or warming and energizing. He says *panax* is better for stimulating sexual activity and other conditions such as poor circulation and digestion and slow metabolisms, especially in older people, while *quinquefolius* is more effective for those who are active, agitated, or nervous, and for young, fit, active people.

The scientific basis for these claims is that all varieties of ginseng have different combinations of a chemical component called ginsenosides. For example, *quinquefolius* has more of Rb1 group ginsenosides, which increase stamina, learning ability, and offset fatigue, insomnia, nervousness, and restlessness. *Panax* has more Rg1 group ginsenosides, which make it more stimulating and arousing.

Is Ginseng Right for Me?

As a naturopathic doctor, I treat each patient as a unique individual. That means each person gets their own individualized treatment plan. All the herbs recommended here can help enhance sexual experience, but it is up to you to work out the best combination based on your own needs and goals. If a person wants to enhance athletic performance, or combat a predisposition to the following conditions, then there is a high probablity the person will benefit from ginseng's combination of actions:

- Anxiety
- Blood sugar control
- Chronic immune challenges (infections, cancer, herpes, etc.)
- Fatigue
- Immune stimulation
- Stress
- Menopausal symptoms

In keeping with the naturopathic principle of prevention, taking ginseng can keep these conditions at bay while enhancing sexual health.

4 WILD OATS

Oats are a wild grain native to the Caspian Sea–Black Sea area of Europe. As a wild grass, this plant grows two to three feet in height depending on the climate and soil conditions. The medicinal components of oats are the ripe seeds and threshed stem and leaf.

Ancient Roots

While "wild oats" are commonly given the botanical name *Avena sativa*, the Latin word *sativa* actually means "cultivated" (according to "Herbal Ed" Smith, founder of HerbPharm). This nutritious grain has been cultivated for about 2,000 years, mostly in Europe and North America. It has both food and medicinal uses. The ground seed becomes oatmeal. The grasses can be cut for tea. Mature, unprocessed oats are called "groats," and the seed husk is ground for oatbran. For herbal medicine, the seed is harvested a little before it matures, while it is in a "milky" state.

Oats have a strong reputation as a nerve tonic that provides deep relaxation. They have been used throughout the centuries to treat conditions such as anxiety, insomnia, stress, and more recently, tobacco and other drug withdrawals. Other medicinal uses include treatment for poor connective tissue tone, gout, kidney and gallbladder disorders, arthritis, constipation, diarrhea, fatigue, and coughs.

Oats also are reputed to be a sexual stimulant in both humans and animals. It is said that horses that eat wild oats are more likely to mate, and with more vigor. As happens sometimes, our very language provides us with reminders of older beliefs and customs; we still uses phrases like, "feeling his oats" and "sowing wild oats."

How It Works

Oats contain numerous chemical constituents, vitamins, and minerals. This grain is a rich source of polysaccharides (complex chains of sugars used by the body for fuel, some of which are also used medically for their immune system stimulation properties) and proteins such as gliadin, avenin, and avenalin. In addition, oats supply steroidal saponins, which some researchers believe influence hormone balances; and beta sitosterol, a plant-based sterol that chemically resembles testosterone, progesterone, and estrogen and is believed to modulate hormonal levels, indirectly and possible directly. Oats also supply alkaloids such as gramine and avenine, fatty acids, and B-vitamins. The seeds are rich in iron, manganese, and zinc, and zinc has been shown to be a vital component of men's sexual and reproductive health. The sterol compounds, like beta sitosterol, and zinc are important nutrients and building blocks that help maintain proper testosterone balance and metabolism, while keeping the tissues healthy, resilient, and responsive throughout the body, including the reproductive tract.

Oats' relaxing effects have been attributed to its alkaloid content. While the exact mechanism has not been determined, alkaloids in other substances such as nicotine, codeine, and cocaine have demonstrated relaxation effects. Feeling relaxed—being in the groove—is crucial to setting the stage for a great sexual encounter. In Chapter One, "The Right Chemistry," we discussed the sabotaging effects of stress on your love life—stress sets in motion a tidal wave of adrenaline and cortisol that puts the damper on your sex drive. The relaxing effect of oats could be just the antidote. The dose of B vitamins from this herb helps fight stress, too.

The humble oat is indeed a powerful medicine. It also epitomizes the concept of food as your best medicine, a concept I mentioned in the introduction to this book as being a keystone of naturopathic medical philosophy.

Research: Sexy Results

While there are volumes of research on the nutritional effects of oats—it helps lower cholesterol, prevent cancer, lower triglycerides, and other wonderful things—I could find little research on the reputed sexual effects of oats. The main source is the Institute for Advanced Study of Human Sexuality in San Francisco, where Ted McIlvenna, Ph.D., began research on the sexual enhancing properties of oats in 1976. Research at the institute has demonstrated that oats have dramatic aphrodisiac effects.

In 1986, the institute conducted a study of men and women who had complaints ranging from impotence, lack of desire, and inability to respond optimally to sexual stimuli, to merely lamenting that they needed to spice up their sex lives. Of those who were given a wild oats formula as part of this research project, the reported effects included heightened sexual awareness, increased sexual feeling and sexual thoughts, even more orgasms: 36 percent more in men and 29 percent more in women, with women also reporting a 68 percent increase in multiple orgasms.

This initial study spurred a more comprehensive double-blind crossover study, which reported the following results: A large portion of the men experienced increased sex drive, firmer erections, and increased sexual pleasure when taking the wild oats formula compared to the placebo (dummy pill). Women reported increased sexual desire, increased sexual fantasy, and more vigorous pursuit of sexual fulfillment.

Of the study participants, three men and three women were selected from the second study group to have their hormone levels checked; all of the women and one of the men had no changes in hormone levels. However, two of the men who earlier had below-normal testosterone levels demonstrated dramatic increases in these levels, at least double their pre-study amounts. These two men also reported powerful sexual changes: One man increased his sexual activity by three to six times over his earlier level of activity; the other man, who had been impotent for six years, went from no activity to being sexually active one to three times a week.

Dr. McIlvenna attributes this dramatic increase in sex drive to an enzyme in the plant that helps unbind testosterone from other substances in the body (for example, sometimes as people age, testosterone will bind to proteins), freeing it to increase libido in both men and women. "This formula gives a man the same interest in sex he had at 14," Dr. McIlvenna said. He cautions that only a concentrated formula delivers these results. "You could eat 15,000 oats and you wouldn't feel a thing."

Patti Britton, Ph.D., certified sex therapist and one of Dr. McIlvenna's clinical research partners, said she has been working with patients taking his formula and noted their reported responses. "I've seen the results dramatically effect sexual energy and desire in both men and women," Dr. Britton said. She said the formula that Dr. McIlvenna developed increases libido and intensifies sexual sensation especially in the glans, or tip, of the penis. Women also experienced increased libido, as well as increased lubrication, leading her to speculate that something in oats also acts on estrogen activity.

Fast Action

Dr. Patti Britton, a certified sex therapist, said she has seen Dr. McIlvenna's oat formula (Vigorex is the commercial name—Forte for men and Femme for women) work very quickly to increase libido. "In my own research with women, the results have showed up in as little as three hours." She told the story of a 30-year-old married woman with a year-old child who lost her interest in sex during her postpartum depression. "She had zero libido," Dr. Britton said. "Her husband brought her to see me out of desperation. Within three hours, it (the Vigorex) kicked in. She called him at work and said, 'Come home, come home!' That's not an unusual report."

 She also told of a 45-year-old married woman with a history of gynecological problems who also had lost her sexual desire. "Within a day her libido was restored," Dr. Britton said, and the woman reported that this product changed her life.

With results like this, Dr. Britton cautioned, Vigorex is nothing to toy with. "This is not something one should take lightly as a road for sexual happiness," she said. "You should have sexual outlet, a regular partner or self-pleasure; the ambience needs to be appropriate."

Side Effects

There are no reported side effects from oats unless a person is sensitive or allergic to them as a food source, or to gluten.

A study conducted on mice demonstrated that oats may reduce the pain-relieving benefits of morphine.

Not for Everyone

People who suffer from gluten or gliadin sensitivity should avoid eating oats. Gluten is a protein derivative of oats, wheat, and other grains (barley, rye, and spelt) that gives the bread dough made from these grains a tough, elastic quality. Gliadin is a chemical component of gluten.

Some physicians believe that persons suffering from celiac disease (a gluten sensitivity that irritates the intestines and results in diarrhea, rashes, bloating, and fatigue) should not come in contact either internally or externally with oats. It can increase the dermatitis (an irritating skin condition) that can accompany this disease.

The Formula That Works

Researchers used a particular commercial formula of wild oats in their studies. The dosages listed below range widely; you can start at the low end and work your way up.

Tea:
One tablespoon of oats per cup of water can be consumed 2–4 times a day

Capsules/Tablets:
1000 mg, 3–4 times a day

Tincture (Alcohol extract):
30–60 drops, 3–4 times a day

As a side note, 150–200 grams of oats (1–2 cups) can be used in a bath to relieve itching from eczema, poison ivy and poison oak.

Are Oats Right for Me?

Unless you are allergic to oats, or sensitive to gluten or gliadin as is the case with celiac sufferers, oats are a great addition to your diet. In fact, this food sounds almost too good to be true: It can lower your cholesterol, relax you, help you sleep, and possibly help you break your smoking habit. Its fiber may lessen the chance of getting certain types of cancer, including colon cancer and certain estrogen dependent cancers, as well. Who couldn't use this kind of help? Start munching!

5 YOHIMBE

Yohimbe, an evergreen tree native to the West African countries of Congo, Cameroon, and Gabon, is the only herb listed in the Physician's Desk Reference as supporting sexual function. Its reputation was upheld by no less authority than the U.S. Food and Drug Administration, which approved Yohimbine as the first plant-derived drug proven in the treatment of impotence, years before Viagra came along.

Yohimbe's Latin name is *Pausinystalia yohimbe* (also referred to as *Corynanthe yohimbe*). The tree grows as high as 85 feet, and its bark is the medicinal part used by the indigenous people to enhance their sexual experience. Yohimbe bark is a gray-brown color, and is frequently discolored by spots. The bark often splits to reveal a red hue underneath.

Ancient Roots

Yohimbe has been used for centuries to treat leprosy, coughs, and fevers among native West Africans. Other conditions treated with yohimbe include weakness and fatigue. Of course, its strong aphrodisiac properties did not go unnoticed for long, and the indigenous people probably began to use the bark even when they weren't ill, to intensify their sexual encounters.

Europeans discovered this natural aphrodisiac about 75 years ago and it has been used widely in Western Europe ever since.

How It Works

Called "herbal Viagra" by the February 1999 edition of *Environmental Nutrition*, yohimbe's power comes from a combination of alkaloids. Alkaloids are organic plant substances that have strong medicinal properties and are frequently used as drugs. Chemically speaking, alkaloids must contain at least one nitrogen molecule. Some potent alkaloids you already know about are cocaine, nicotine, morphine, quinine, and codeine.

Among yohimbe's alkaloids that possess medicinal properties is one called yohimbine (from which the brand-name pharmaceutical version derives its name), ajamalicin, corynathein, and dihydrocorynanethein. The alkaloid yohimbine blocks alpha–2-adrenergic nerve activity, which normally constricts the blood vessels. By blocking this nerve activity, vessels are allowed to dilate. The result is that yohimbe increases blood flow, while reducing blood pressure. As we have mentioned in earlier chapters, increased blood flow means the ability to get erections is enhanced.

Another effect of the alkaloid yohimbine is that it acts as a monoamine oxidase (MAO) inhibitor. Monoamine oxidase is an enzyme (hence the ending -ase), that destroys adrenaline and neurotransmitters like serotonin that send and receive messages in the brain. Inhibiting the MAOs results in an increase in neurotransmitters, so your brain is sending and receiving more clearly; that's why prescription drugs for depression often use MAO inhibiting action. Though yohimbe may show some promise in this direction, the scientific research has not been conducted using this herb for depression. Just consider that the mood-elevating properties of yohimbe are a positive side effect when the herb is used carefully to boost libido and performance.

Recently, scientists also have found that yohimbe may aid in weight loss by suppressing the body's ability to store fat. This may be caused by the same mechanism that blocks the nerve activity that constricts blood vessels. Since weight loss has not, so far, been a major use of yohimbe, there hasn't been any research into how this actually works, and for this reason I would not recommend yohimbe as a weight-loss treatment. I can tell you, though, that I have had patients who experienced substantial weight loss while taking yohimbe, more than could be accounted for from increased sexual activity, and without dietary changes.

More Sex, Less Weight

Generally speaking, most of the literature generally infers that women should avoid use of yohimbe. I have not seen this substantiated in my clinical experience, although I would not recommend it for a pregnant or nursing woman. But under other conditions, yohimbe works to increase libido and sexual gratification for women as well.

For example, one of my patients, a 28-year-old woman, reported taking yohimbe for six months to heighten her sexual experience. The form she used was a prescribed standardized concentrated tincture (liquid in an alcohol base) of 15 mg twice a day. She said she experienced increased desire as well as more intense orgasms, and was very pleased to have lost 50 pounds in the bargain.

This is a very aggressive weight loss and it is not without risk. This is because our fat stores toxins such as pesticides from our food and air, and waste byproducts from cellular activity. Releasing that kind of toxic burden so quickly can actually harm the body, since the liver must process all those released chemicals. One way to guard against an overworked liver in this case, or in general, is to drink lots of water, take antioxidants, and eat lots of fiber to bind up the toxins.

Research: Sexy Results

Since research on yohimbe was aimed at getting FDA approval for treatment of impotence, most studies were conducted on men who were totally unable to achieve an erection. Traditional and clinical use, however, confirm yohimbe's action in healthy people to increase libido and performance. Research such as that cited here upholds my observation that patients who take yohimbe benefit from an overall boost to sexual performance as well as recovery of some loss of function.

- A recent review of more than half a dozen well-controlled clinical trials showed yohimbine more effective than a placebo on treating erectile dysfunction of both physical and psychological origin.

- Researchers in a Stanford University study isolated the exact level of yohimbe from the bark of an African tree long reputed to be an aphrodisiac. This study found subjects experienced a 90 percent increase in sexual desire in less than one hour.

- In a double-blind study conducted for the United States Veterans Administration, 182 men with erectile dysfunction took 42 mg of oral yohimbine hydrochloride (the pharmaceutical drug form) daily. The subjects' health problems included diabetes and cardiovascular problems, both of which diminish circulation, and as we discussed in Chapter 1: The Right Chemistry, circulation is critical to sexual functioning. Even with these serious conditions, 14 percent experienced complete restoration of full and sustained erections within one month, and another 20 percent reported partial response. As reported in the medical journal *Urology*, subjects in the study reported that the maximal effect of the drug is experienced within 2–3 weeks.

Otherwise healthy individuals should experience substantially better results than this study's response rate of 34 percent, particularly if all the equipment is in good working order, which was not the case in these study participants. I ask all my patients to list the supplements they are taking, and I often see yohimbe on the list of those who have not reported any sexual difficulties. The men say it helps them get more substantial and rigid erections, and that it enhances not only their libido but overall sexual sensations.

- Yohimbe also works for men who have some psychological reason for their inability to achieve an erection. In a double-blind study of 48 men with psychogenic impotence, 46 percent of the men reported improvement in sexual functioning. The conclusion of this study, reported in the British medical journal *Lancet*, was that yohimbine could be a safe adjunct to sex and marital therapy for improving sexual satisfaction.

- A subject in one study reported that not only was his sex life improving, so was his narcolepsy. In a followup study, seven out of eight people were able to stay awake for a normal eight-hour shift. Researchers suspect it may counteract the brain chemistry that causes narcolepsy. Study author Virgil Wooten, M.D., associate professor of internal medicine at Eastern Virginia Medical School, said yohimbe gives promise of being more effective than the current medication for narcolepsy, without the negative side effects of the treatment now used (and with one rather positive side effect—something worth staying awake for!).

First Things First

A 53-year-old man came to my office looking for a remedy that would help him maintain an erection. While he had no trouble feeling aroused, he simply couldn't stay erect, and both he and his partner were frustrated.

As a naturopathic doctor, I always want to deal with the causes first, and in this case the cause was initial stage of benign prostatic hyperplasia (BPH), swelling of the prostate that diminishes circulation to the sex organs. But herbal remedies can take a month or more to begin to see improvement in BPH, and several months to achieve a significant effect. I knew my patient needed a boost immediately to keep him with the program. A standardized form of yohimbe from his local pharmacy was just the ticket.

Within three weeks, he was reporting more substantial and sustained erections. After a few months, we added saw palmetto, which helped lessen his prostate enlargement and helped relieve the cause of his trouble.

Side Effects

While yohimbe has demonstrated great success on increasing libido and improving sexual performance, there are many cautions to using this botanical remedy. These were recognized by the FDA, which placed yohimbe on the "unsafe herb" list. Many herbs and pharmaceutical compounds pose a hazard to our health if not used properly—

just read the small print on any over-the-counter cold or sinus remedy. But like those medicines, actual health hazards have not been noted when yohimbe is prescribed correctly for individuals at appropriate dosages.

Among the more frequent side effects mentioned in research are increased blood pressure, nausea and/or vomiting, insomnia, racing heart, tremor, and anxiety. Others may experience headache, irritability, or muscle aches. At high enough doses, hallucinations have been reported, but do not try this at home, folks; this is no recreational drug. If hallucinations occur, discontinue usage at once. Overdose can result in heart irregularity that can lead to death for those in delicate health. Other possible symptoms include dilation of the pupils, diarrhea, low blood pressure due to heart disturbance, and excess salivation.

After reading the above paragraph, you may find it contradictory that yohimbe can trigger both lower blood pressure and higher blood pressure. Here's how that works. Yohimbe's stimulatory effect pushes up blood pressure in the short term, and as the heart becomes overwhelmed and becomes unable to keep up with demand, pressure starts dropping. It's like when you overwork your biceps at the gym—eventually the muscle stops contracting. When this happens to the heart, blood pressure drops.

No, Thanks!

Yohimbe's stimulatory effect on circulation can be a boon and a bane. Ed Smith, life-long herbalist and founding president of HerbPharm, tells the story of a friend who experimented with yohimbe. He brewed a strong tea from the bark and drank a pint of it. Within half an hour, he had not only a throbbing erection, but a throbbing headache. "With every heartbeat, I hurt in both places," he recalls. "The last thing I wanted was to have sex—I just wanted that erection to go away!"

Not for Everyone

Though yohimbe is available at health food stores, it is a prescription drug, and should be monitored by your physician. Here is a list of conditions that preclude the use of yohimbe:

- Anxiety
- Benign Prostatic Hyperplasia
- Bi-polar disorder
- Depression
- Heart disease
- High blood pressure
- Kidney disease
- Liver disease
- Manic-depressive illness
- Pregnant/breastfeeding women
- Schizophrenia

Yohimbe should not be taken without close doctor supervision, especially if you are taking an antidepressant or a high blood pressure medicine, since it can lessen the effectiveness of these medications, and may increase the risk of negative side effects. Alcohol also may decrease the effectiveness of yohimbe while increasing the risk of side effects.

There is also some theoretical concern about ingesting large amounts of tyramine when using yohimbe regularly. Tyramine is formed in decaying or matured foods; overripe bananas and avocados are notable sources of this substance. Cured and smoked foods also contain tyramine, which is structurally very close to adrenaline and has similar, but weaker, stimulant effects. Eating one overripe banana while taking yohimbe probably would not cause a problem for most people as long as they are not also taking any type of anti-depressant; nevertheless, if a person ate a lot of these foods on a regular basis, or ate a large quantity in one sitting, theoretically an interaction with yohimbe could occur. Given yohimbe's stimulating properties, it's best not to mix this adrenaline-like chemical with the herb, which may lead to a temporary spike of high blood pressure.

If you are taking any medication, particularly the following drugs, you should consult your physician before trying yohimbe.

- Allergy medication (especially those containing ephedrine and pseudoephedrine)
- Amobarbital
- Atropine
- Beta blockers
- Clonidine
- Epinephrine
- Guanabenz
- MAO inhibitors
- Methylnorepinephrine
- Naloxone
- Phenothiazines
- Phenoxybenzamine
- Phentolamine
- Reserpine
- Tricyclic antidepressants

The Formula That Works

The principal form of yohimbe is the alkaloid yohimbine hydrochloride. You can look it up by this name in any book about prescription drugs or the Physicians Desk Reference (PDR). Common brand names for prescription-strength yohimbe include: Actibine, Aphrodyne, Baron-X, Dayto, Himbin, Prohim, Thybine, Yocon, Yohimar, Yohimex, Yoman, and YoVital. In this form, you work up to a total of

15–25 milligrams per day, preferably divided into several doses, with or without food. Doses as high as 40 milligrams can increase effectiveness; however, these dosage levels definitely warrant medical supervision. Even at lower doses, yohimbe can cause serious side effects in susceptible individuals.

Yohimbe also comes in a tincture form, that is, a concentrated herbal formula in an alcohol base, administered by dropper. The dosage in tincture form varies greatly; follow the directions given on the package. Your best bet is to start the use of this, and other forms of yohimbe, in an incremental fashion. Typically, doses are started at the low end and a therapeutic range is worked up to for each individual over the course of 3–4 weeks.

The clinical effectiveness of yohimbe is dependent on its yohimbine content. At the correct dose, yohimbe can add a spark to your sex life. It should be noted that the products available in most health food stores across the United States vary greatly in terms of active ingredients and finding a standardized product is crucial, especially given yohimbe's possible side effects. Look for products that say the formula is standardized. That means there is quality control to ensure the amount of active ingredient is the same in every dose. A company that claims its products are standardized will be able to produce a certificate of analysis, which you can obtain through your health food department or store manager, although this may require some persistence. Since the U.S. Food and Drug Administration does not regulate herbs, it is up to the consumer to look for and insist upon quality standardized products. In one of the appendices, you will find a list of self-policing organizations that promote quality control in the supplement industry.

Is Yohimbe Right for Me?

Healthy men and women in their 20s to 50s should be able to use yohimbe in moderate doses to enhance their sexual enjoyment, although I recommend they get a full physical and their doctor's okay beforehand. I can't recommend yohimbe for older adults for two reasons: 1) It hasn't been tested extensively on them, and 2) it's too risky, given a person's potentially declining health (diagnosed or not) during these years and the herb's potential negative side effects. However, if your health will withstand the increased blood supply to your sex organs and potentially increased blood pressure, and you have none of the listed conditions and take none of the mentioned medications, you may enjoy the tremendous benefits of increased libido, heightened sexual sensations and improved performance.

6 ESPECIALLY FOR MEN

In cultures around the world, from ancient times to the present, healers have characterized some herbs as "male" and others as "female" because of their apparent gender-specific actions. In fact, we do find there are herbs that provide gender-specific benefits, and in "Especially for Men," we'll examine several of them and explain their contributions to men's reproductive health and sexual performance.

The Forgotten Sex Organ

Key to your performance, of course, is keeping all the equipment in good shape. I imagine, though, that your prostate is not the first organ you think of when it comes to your sexual equipment, or even the second. Think again—researchers believe sensations that occur in this walnut-sized organ during ejaculation heighten orgasmic feelings. The prostate also makes vital contributions to your sperm function. These two features ought to earn the prostate some respect, yet it is chiefly known as something that makes it difficult for "older" men to urinate (have you noticed that however old you are, "older" always means someone else?). It takes many years for the prostate to enlarge to the point of causing serious problems, yet, even by age 30, about 10 percent of men demonstrate noticeable signs of prostate enlargement. That's one out of 10 men. Unfortunately, your chances of having early prostate symptoms are a whole lot better than hitting the lottery.

Not all the prostate's functions are understood. It acts as both a gland and an accessory sex organ; the prostate secretes some of the fluids that make up semen and also contracts during orgasm. Running right through the prostate are ducts leading from the seminal vesicles (a repository for mature sperm) and from the bladder. These join to become the urethra, which ends at the tip of the penis and carries urine and sperm. When the prostate enlarges, and it can grow to be the size of a small orange, it puts the squeeze on the urethra. This hampers urine flow and can dampen the libido and sexual performance, too.

The "early warning system" for prostate enlargement is difficulty urinating. How's your stream? Can you still blast a tin can at six paces? If you are noticing changes, that's a hallmark symptom of benign prostatic hyperplasia (BPH) and other prostate changes warranting attention. The stream doesn't flow like it used to, not as strongly, not as quickly, not as focused. That's because abnormal hormone action, which I'll describe a little later, tricks your prostate into enlarging. In fact, the prostate can make itself two or three times larger than normal before you even get a diagnosis. As BPH advances, you feel like you have to urinate all the time, and never feel quite done.

The symptoms of BPH are so stereotypical that even movies make fun of them without realizing what they signify. George Segal and Richard Benjamin, in *The Last Married Couple in America,* are in the men's room and Benjamin's character is in a frenzy of despair because his "stream" isn't as strong as it used to be and he feels that it symbolizes his entire life. In *Wrestling Ernest Hemingway,* Robert Duvall and Richard Harris play a couple of old guys who, in one scene, are urinating into a stream that reflects Fourth of July fireworks. As they stand there—and stand there—in that unmistakable pose against the blazing night sky, Harris turns to Duvall and says, "Remember when this didn't take so long?"

If you are having any of these symptoms, square your shoulders and check in with your urologist. There are a lot worse things than the rubber glove exam (take my word for it—I'm a doctor!). If you are over 40, a simple blood test called a PSA (prostate specific antigen) is highly recommended by many doctors and can give you vital information on the health of your prostate.

One current standard medical treatment for BPH is a drug called finasteride; the most popular prescribed version is called Proscar. The good news is that this drug works well for alleviating the symptoms of BPH; the bad news is that its side effects may include loss of libido and impotence. According to the journal *Patient Care,* the U.S. Food and Drug Administration may be on the brink of approving the use of saw palmetto, the first herb we discuss in this chapter, for treatment of BPH. The good news is that, according to some studies, saw palmetto has been clinically proven to be as effective as finasteride for alleviating symptoms; the great news is that this herb enhances both libido and performance instead of diminishing them. As if this weren't enough, saw palmetto does all this for a fraction of the cost of the prescription drug, and the herb is readily available in standardized forms.

Aside from BPH, the most common male complaint is prostatitis, a bacterial or viral infection that usually stems from a urinary tract infection. This condition is treated conventionally with antibiotics; I have successfully treated it with immune-stimulating nutrients and with herbs that have specific prostate benefits, like those we discuss in this chapter. Prostatitis can be the result of a sexually transmitted disease, but it doesn't have to be, so don't give your partner the evil eye if this happens to you. Stress and dehydration are two other culprits. A symptom of dehydration is deeper urine color; if you are getting enough water, it should be a pale straw color. Prostatitis manifests with symptoms similar to BPH. Either of these conditions can wreak havoc on your sleep, not to mention your sexual desire. So watch for the first signs, the urinary changes, to safeguard your sex life and overall wellbeing.

The herbs we examine in this chapter can not only treat, but can help to prevent prostate disease because they address the underlying causes. Several of them have centuries of practical application, as well as recent research, to substantiate their effects. Saw palmetto and pygeum decrease the chemical interaction that results in an enlarged prostate, and they have antiseptic and anti-microbial effects that guard against infection. Plant pollen and stinging nettles offer similar benefits for prostate health. Even if you can still nail a tin can at six paces, you've got to be intrigued by an herb dubbed "potency wood" by Brazilian natives who take muira puama to get as hard as the tree whose bark they use. We'll close the chapter with a few tips for men's sexual health that go beyond herbs to lifestyle factors such as food and beer.

SAW PALMETTO

Called *Serenoa repens* (sometimes *Serenoa serrulata*), saw palmetto is a scrubby little tree native to a narrow strip paralleling the Atlantic seaboard from South Carolina to Florida. It also grows in coastal Southern California. These trees can live to be centuries old, but they seldom get taller than 6–10 feet high. They are crowned with a three-foot-wide fan of long, spiky leaves. The oblong berries are about $1/2$ to 1 inch long and grow in a cluster weighing up to nine pounds. The berries' color can be red, deep brown, or even black. Their taste is said to be somewhat sweet, but not pleasant, and they contain a hard brown seed. After ripening, the berries can be partially dried and used as medicine.

Ancient Roots

Native Americans have used the berries of the saw palmetto to treat urinary and reproductive tract imbalances since at least the 1700s. It was believed that the berry increased sperm production and sex drive in men. They used it to increase testicular functions and support the health of the prostate. Women also found some use for it, eating the berries to help disorders of the breast, and even to enlarge the breasts. Saw palmetto berry also has long been upheld as an aphrodisiac by many herbalists, according to James Duke, Ph.D., in his *Handbook of Medicinal Herbs*.

In the early part of this century, saw palmetto berry tea was commonly recommended by clinicians for benign enlargement of the prostate. It was also used to treat chronic urinary tract infections. Although it lost favor in the U.S., it is still used widely in Europe.

In addition to these sex-related actions, saw palmetto has other medicinal uses. It acts as a diuretic, a sedative, and a tonic. Historically, it was also used as a decongestant for treating respiratory infections.

How It Works

Most of the chemically active ingredients of saw palmetto are fatty acids and similar compounds called lipid sterols. Among the fatty acids are caprylic acid, lauric acid, palmitic acid, and oleic acid (also found in olive oil), which have an antiseptic effect. Beyond these fatty acids, saw palmetto berries serve up a cornucopia of nutrients: They are a rich source of carotenes, a form of vitamin A found particularly in red, orange, and yellow vegetables, such as carrots, which also have anti-oxidant properties; tannins, which are anti-microbial agents also found in teas; and lipase, a digestive enzyme that helps break down fat. The presence of lipase is an example of nature's inherent balance: The berries are high in fat, and lipase is supplied to help the body digest the fat.

The most prevalent clinical use of saw palmetto is the treatment of benign prostate hyperplasia (BPH). I mentioned earlier in this chapter that the prostate can be tricked into enlarging itself. Here's how that works. Dihydrotestosterone (DHT), one of several forms of testosterone, can bind to receptor sites on the membranes of prostate cells and their nuclei. Too much DHT can cause the prostate cells to divide and multiply at a higher-than-normal rate, leading to an enlargement of the gland. The fatty acids in saw palmetto combat this powerful form of male hormone, first by limiting the conversion of normal testosterone to DHT, then by preventing DHT from binding to prostate cells and triggering excess growth.

Advanced BPH is one of the leading factors in less-than-firm erections as men age. Although BPH is more prevalent in men over 45, younger men may also notice subtle changes in their ability to perform. If your bladder feels full because an enlarged prostate is pushing against it, it is difficult to keep your mind on the situation at hand. The pressure that arises from BPH detracts from the inner tension that many men say they feel during arousal and ejaculation. In this way, BPH can detract not only from your sexual performance, but from your sexual pleasure as well.

Research: Sexy Results

Saw palmetto is another wonderful instance of scientific research validating traditional herbal medicine, and in this case, research shows it is even more effective than conventional medical treatment. Numerous studies have shown saw palmetto to be effective in 90 percent of patients suffering from BPH within the first year of treatment, compared to a success rate of less than 50 percent for patients taking finasteride, one of the most commonly prescribed drugs, for this condition.

Researchers led by Timothy J. Wilt, M.D., M.P.H., and director of a group that studies prostate diseases for the Minnesota Veterans Affairs Medical Center, conducted a systematic review of saw palmetto in more than a dozen European studies performed in the past three decades and encompassing nearly 3,000 men. Their findings, published in the November 1998 issue of the *Journal of the American Medical Association*, support the use of saw palmetto for BPH. "Compared with finasteride, *S repens* (saw palmetto) produces similar improvements in urinary tract symptoms, has fewer adverse treatment effects and costs less," the authors concluded.

One of the studies Dr. Wilt and his colleagues reviewed was a multi-center study designed by J. Braekman and published in the *Journal of Current Therapeutic Research*, 1994. More than 300 men suffering from classic BPH-related urination symptoms took 160 milligrams of saw palmetto two times a day. At the 45-day mark, 83 percent of the men reported that the herb offered effective relief of symptoms; at 90 days, the percentage increased to 88 percent.

In one double-blind study, as Daniel B. Mowrey, Ph.D., reports in his *Herbal Tonic Therapies*, saw palmetto was given to 100 patients suffering from BPH. The frequency of getting up during the night to urinate decreased by more than 45 percent, the rate of urine flow increased by more than 50 percent, and the residual urine (left in the bladder because of insufficient pressure to get past the prostate's blockage of the urethra) decreased by 42 percent in the treatment group.

"Saw palmetto extract, concentrated and purified in the best tradition of guaranteed potency herbs, dramatically reduces the size of the enlarged prostate and restores function," Mowrey says.

Because of saw palmetto's wonderful preventative action—keeping DHT from triggering the increase of prostate cells—if you start taking it early, there's a good chance you may forestall prostate enlargement, and the symptoms that can put the breaks on your love life.

What's My Prostate Got to Do with My Sex Life?

Ryan thought prostate problems were for old guys. He was feeling pretty fit and healthy in his mid-40s, with plenty of libido but faulty equipment. "What's my prostate got to do with sex, anyway?" he asked.

Ryan initially came to see me because he was having increasing difficulty urinating. His medical doctor diagnosed benign prostate hyperplasia and put him on the accepted prescription drug, Proscar. Ryan took the medication for six months but he was still having to urinate 2–3 times a night, and couldn't get what he called a "meaningful erection."

I recommended a product that contained saw palmetto extract, pygeum, and pumpkin seed extract. He was very happy with the results—within 5 weeks, he was getting up only once a night to urinate and was having much better success with his sexual performance. Ryan's case was advanced, and I have seen an even quicker response to treatment in men who didn't wait as long as he did to take action.

Side Effects

Studies and human clinical trials have demonstrated that saw palmetto can be taken safely for long periods of time with no negative side effects. I could find no reports of risks associated with using saw palmetto.

Not for Everyone

A search of the relevant scientific literature turned up no references to negative drug interactions or health conditions that preclude the use of saw palmetto. There is one caution, however. Some doctors think saw palmetto interferes with an accurate Prostate Specific Antigen (PSA) test for BPH. Clinically speaking, it makes sense that saw palmetto should lower PSA scores; it addresses the cause of elevated antigen levels that the test measures. If you are planning to take a PSA test, stop taking your saw palmetto for about two weeks beforehand; that should lessen the likelihood of the herb affecting your test results.

The Formula That Works

Dr. Wilt and his colleagues, who conducted the review of research on saw palmetto for the November 1998 issue of the *Journal of the American Medical Association,* say that their review did not find an established dosage of saw palmetto for the safe treatment of BPH and additional long-term study is required on that point. There are guidelines, however, based on recommendations by doctors and the dosages approved by other countries. For example, the German E Commission, which has reviewed clinical studies of 380 herbs and approved the medicinal use of 254 of them, recommends 1–2 grams of the crude (raw) herb per day. If you want to try the raw herb, it is available at some health food stores. Look for products that specify they are organic or wildcrafted. I suggest to my patients that they take, instead, the standardized extracts available at health food stores, at the German E Commission's recommended dosage of 320 mg a day. This is the same dosage that other clinicians have recommended for their patients taking saw palmetto.

In *Natural Prescriptions,* Robert M. Giller, M.D., reports that saw palmetto has given many of his patients relief from BPH at the 320 mg dosage level.

In *Natural Health, Natural Medicine*, Andrew Weil, M.D., also recommends this dosage. "This remedy protects the prostate from the irritating effects of testosterone and, by promoting shrinkage of the gland, improves urinary function," he says. "It is nontoxic and you can stay on it indefinitely."

When you shop for saw palmetto, be sure to look for a compound that specifies on the label that it has 85–95% fatty acids and liposterols. Also, the powdered dried berry (remember, it is the fruit of this plant that is medicinal) can be taken as a tea. Since this is weaker than the herbal extract, 5–6 grams (about 2 tablespoons) may be taken per day. Liquid extracts of the whole herb at 5–6 ml per day can also be effective.

If you decide to try saw palmetto to relieve BPH, you may not see results for four to six weeks, although some men report an immediate improvement. In my practice, I have waited as long as 120 days to hear a positive report from my patients, so try not to be impatient. If you have an improvement, the saw palmetto can be continued. It may be that the improvement is so gradual, you may not realize it at first. While saw palmetto has little immediate effect, it does have the ability to change actual biochemical interactions in the body. As mentioned earlier, the herb allows testosterone function to be modulated and directed to pathways that support health by preventing the conversion of normal testosterone to DHT, which, when left unchecked, leads to prostate enlargement and diminished sexual function.

Is Saw Palmetto Right for Me?

If you are a guy of any age, but especially in your 40s or above, and you have noticed that your ability to urinate has changed, check for these common symptoms of a growing prostate.

- Hesitancy when urinating (You just can't get started, despite urgent feelings.)

- Forked stream (Your ability to hit the target has decreased.)

- Increased frequency (Wasn't I here just a minute ago?)

- Nighttime trips (How is a guy to get any sleep?)

- Incomplete voiding (Come on, I know there is more!)

When you start having symptoms like these, a good preventative measure is to get yourself tested. Even if no BPH shows up on the test, try some saw palmetto and see if the symptoms abate.

MUIRA PUAMA

An herb that goes by the name of "potency wood" must have a solid reputation, and this rain forest remedy lives up to its nickname. Muira puama is a staple of Amazonian folk medicine, and is best known as an aphrodisiac. M. Penna, in his 1930 book *Notas Sobre Plantas Brasileiras (Notes on Brazilian Plants)*, wrote that, "Marapuama has long been valued as an aphrodisiac and tonic for the nervous system."

European explorers took it home with them and it has long been listed in the conservative British Herbal Pharmacopoeia, which reluctantly acknowledges muira puama's aphrodisiac action, recommending it to treat impotence. Although it has been known for hundreds of years and has been used widely in Europe and South America, muira puama has yet to gain a firm following in the U.S.

Muira puama grows in Brazil's Amazon rain forest and in neighboring Guyana, presenting another reason to not destroy one of nature's richest pharmacies. The tree grows from 15–45 feet tall, bearing white flowers nearly an inch long with a jasmine-like scent. It also produces a fruit that begins with a green coloration that turns pink, then ripens into a light purple color. Historically, almost every part of the tree has been used for food and medicine, but healers focused primarily on the bark and roots. According to some ancient traditions, including those of medieval Europe, the physical characteristics of a plant are assumed to indicate its medicinal value, so perhaps the deep vertical grooves in muira puama's trunk gave the indigenous people a clue to its best and highest use.

Ancient Roots

Folklore throughout South America strongly supports muira puama's stimulating properties. It is commonly referred to not only as an aphrodisiac but also as a nerve stimulant that is said to heighten the receptiveness to sexual stimuli, as well as the physical sensations of sex. If you don't have any trouble with that, you still might want to consider muira puama because of another traditional use; it is a preventative for baldness, according to Steven C. Hollifield, Ac.Phys., in *Healing Forest*.

Native peoples of Brazil also steeped the roots and bark to make a tea that was taken to treat rheumatism, strengthen the heart, and promote intestinal health. They even bathed in it to treat paralysis.

How It Works

Muira puama seems to have two effects: increasing libido and increasing penile hardness. First, let's look at how it may affect libido. Muira puama is rich in naturally occurring sterols, which we have described already as possible building blocks for hormones such as testosterone. Muira puama contains beta sitosterol, campesterol, and also lupeol, another chemical that helps create hormones. Some scientists theorize that beta sitosterol activates the body's receptors for hormones such as testosterone, revving our hormonal engines and leading to both heightened libido and enhanced performance. Also present are numerous other chemicals and volatile oils like camphor, which helps restore the sex drive and inner depth of libido, and other as-yet unidentified constituents. These chemically active components enhance mental ability to become sexually aroused and stimulate nerves to carry messages to pleasure centers in the brain. This action may work as well for women as men, although there doesn't seem to be any folklore or research on muira puama for women.

Regarding muira puama's second hallmark effect, increased penile hardness, this may stem from its apparent effect on circulation. Although researchers are not quite sure how this mechanism works, some are convinced muira puama does help men achieve better erections. Dr. Jacques Waynberg of the Institute of Sexology in Paris called muira puama one of the best herbs for supporting optimal male sexual performance. It sets itself apart, to a degree, because it appears to trigger not only improved penile hardness, but also helps the mind paint a backdrop for more enjoyable and satisfying sex.

Research: Sexy Results

Muira puama has been studied sporadically by researchers in Brazil, France, England, Germany, Japan, and the U.S. for the past eight decades. An article published in a Brazilian pharmacology journal in 1925 recounted a study of muira puama by Rudolpho Dias Da Silva that showed it is an effective treatment for nervous system disorders, impotence, rheumatism, and partial paralysis. M. Penna, in his 1930 book on the folk uses of Amazon herbs, cited clinical experiments conducted in France by a Dr. Rebourgeon confirming muira puama as effective for gastrointestinal complaints, circulation, and impotence.

More recently, J. Waynberg reported the results of his clinical study at the First International Congress on Ethnopharmacology in 1990. In this study, 262 men who complained of low libido and iffy erections took 1000 to 1500 mg of muira puama extract per day. Within two weeks (this is relatively fast action, in naturopathic time!), 62 percent of the men who reported low libido and 51 percent of men with a prior inability to have an erection reported dynamic effects.

Researchers have concluded that, in addition to muira puama's libido-enhancing action on the hormones, it also acts on the nervous system and circulation to prime both a man's psychological and physical ability to enjoy sexual encounters. Certainly, every man wants his equipment optimally ready and, with our stressful lives, a little help in getting those mental engines going is a welcome addition to this herb's action.

Side Effects

In the decades that researchers have been studying muira puama, and in the centuries that it has been used by people around the world, neither folk nor scientific literature have reported any known negative side effects.

Not for Everyone

The literature does not report any level at which toxicity is observed, or any known negative interactions to muira puama.

Muira Puama to the Rescue

With muira puama's overall safety record, it is one of the foremost choices for an otherwise healthy man who wants to intensify moments of intimacy and perform at his peak. Alone or in combination formulas with ginseng or saw palmetto, muira puama and yohimbe are some of my favorite potency potions to prescribe.

It worked well for Alan, who had a high personal performance standard: "Well, see, doc, I used to be able to have sex twice a day, if I wanted to, and still be ready for more action." Alan was luckier than a lot of men I have known, but by the time he came to me in his early 40s, he said his erections weren't as firm as they used to be, and he couldn't keep up the pace anymore. Given his perspective, I asked him what his goal was—increased hardness or increased frequency. He said he would take quality over quantity, because he felt this was more important to his partner.

 I sent him home with a muira puama product and instructed him to avoid sex for one week, then track his level of satisfaction both mentally and physically. Alan wasn't sure about the abstinence part of the assignment, but he was ready to give it a try.

He discussed the issue with his partner, for which he deserves a lot of credit—many men would rather eat dirt. This communication confirmed what he suspected, that his partner really did not feel like sex twice a day and that she would rather focus on quality of experience than notching the bedpost. The bottom line is, they both got what they wanted: Alan felt like his old—or, rather, young—self again and his partner was happy with the results.

The Formula That Works

The dosage used in studies on muira puama is 250 mg, 3 times a day, in capsule form. Research supports using a 6:1 concentrate (meaning the concentrate is six times stronger than the raw herb), so be sure to look for that ratio on the label. No information is available on use of the raw bark, and since we can't be sure of its source, it is best to choose a standardized formula from a reputable supplement manufacturer (see Appendix 2 for suggestions).

Is Muira Puama Right for Me?

Muira puama has been shown to enhance both physical and psychological enjoyment of sex, and that sounds right for everyone. With no known toxicity levels and no observed negative interactions or side effects, it would appear that any man may use muira puama to enhance his sexual performance and experience. If you are taking prescription drugs that affect your circulation or nervous system, start out with lower doses and work up to 250 mg, 3 times a day, paying careful attention to your body's reaction. As with any medication, if you notice any symptoms that alarm you, stop taking the medication immediately and consult your physician.

PYGEUM

Pygeum africanum is an evergreen tree native to the higher elevations of central and southern Africa. It grows to heights of up to 150 feet. Its fruit appears like a ripened cherry, although it is not eaten, and its dull gray-brown bark is used for medicinal purposes.

Ancient Roots

Indigenous peoples used the bark to treat urinary tract infections. They first ground or pulverized the bark, then either dissolved it in milk or palm oil, or prepared it as a tea.

How It Works

Pygeum specifically targets the prostate gland, yet its pharmacological activity is broad, as is often the case with botanical remedies. Its most prevalent clinical uses are treating prostatitis, male infertility, impotence, and benign prostatic hyperplasia (BPH).

Research indicates that the lipophilic (fat soluble) components found in the bark possess pygeum's medicinal properties. Seen in this light, the indigenous practice of dissolving the bark in fat-rich milk or palm oil makes biological sense: The fat in either liquid would allow the active ingredients to dissolve into the beverage, resulting in what scientists call "bio-availability" of the chemical components. This ensures that they will be easily absorbed from the gastrointestinal tract.

The lipophilic extract of pygeum bark has three categories of active constituents:

The phytosterols (sterols found in plants, in contrast to animal-based sterols such as cholesterol), including beta sitosterol, have anti-inflammatory effects which are achieved by interfering with the formation of inflammatory prostaglandins, hormones that tend to accumulate in the prostates of men with BPH.

The terpenes in pygeum have an anti-swelling effect. Terpenes are present in many plants that produce fragrant essential oils. You are already familiar with some terpenes: pinene, the principle ingredient in turpentine, and limonene, the essential oil found in oranges and lemons.

The ferulic esters, another chemically active component of pygeum, reduce levels of the hormone prolactin (most commonly associated with female lactation) and prevent the chemical stimulation that occurs between prostate cells and cholesterol. Reducing prolactin and the chemical action of cholesterol in the prostate are important because these substances are key players in the process that fools the prostate into "hyper" production of its cells, resulting in enlargement.

The cumulative effect of these three actions—the anti-inflammatory, the anti-swelling, and the anti-prolactin and cholesterol properties—work together to minimize prostate enlargement, decreasing the likelihood of infection and promoting proper blood flow to, and nerve health of, the whole genital area.

In addition to the effects of the above components of pygeum, this multifaceted herb also has the indirect effect of reducing the body's testosterone levels, through a fatty acid called N-docosanol. To compensate, pygeum is believed to raise adrenal gland production of androgen and other "male" hormones. This hormonal tradeoff can work well for men who are fighting BPH, which, as we have seen, is prompted by testosterone that turns into DHT, triggering the prostate enlargement that can put the brakes on your love life.

Research: Sexy Results

Extensive research on pygeum has been conducted throughout Europe and has included both human clinical trials and animal studies. Almost all the research on the medicinal properties of pygeum has been done on extracts that were concentrated to particular levels of the active ingredients: 14% terpenes, N-docosanol, and beta sitosterol.

More than 20 clinical trials involving more than 600 men in the past 20 years have demonstrated pygeum's beneficial ability to relieve symptoms of BPH.

When it comes to helping make erections even firmer, pygeum has demonstrated its ability as a player. In a study of both urological and sexual effects of pygeum on men with BPH, Dr. C. Carani reported in an Italian medical journal in 1991 that subjects taking the herb experienced stronger nighttime erections.

Side Effects

In clinical studies, there were very rare reports of mild gastrointestinal irritation in some patients taking pygeum, but no more-serious side effects. There is no known toxicity associated with its proper use.

Not for Everyone

When taken correctly, pygeum is considered one of the safest herbs used for male health. There are no observed negative interactions with other herbs or drugs.

The Formula That Works

The crude dried bark of pygeum (that is, not concentrated or standardized in any way) has not been studied sufficiently to recommend a dose. That's probably okay, since there aren't too many pygeum trees around for us to harvest the bark. Fortunately, there are standardized formulas available in capsule and tablet form. Be sure to check the label for the formula that has been shown effective: standardized 14% terpenes, including beta sitosterol, and .5% N-docosanol. You can take 100–250 mg per day in two separate doses.

The accepted form of pygeum used in Europe for treatment of BPH is a lipophilic extract standardized to 13% total sterols (typically calculated as beta sitosterol). The recommended dose is 50–100 mg, 2 times per day. If you have been diagnosed with BPH, allow 4–8 weeks to notice appreciable results. For those men seeking a tune-up, look for increased erectile strength within about 4 weeks.

Pygeum is also available as a tincture (a liquid form with an alcohol base), but the capsule form is more likely to have standardization of the active ingredients, and this is what I recommend to my patients.

Many experts believe that taking pygeum with saw palmetto offers a high level of synergy and that better and more rapid results can be achieved taking them together. One of my colleagues, Steven Sandberg-Lewis, N.D., said his patients have been very happy with their success using saw palmetto and pygeum together. "I've had patients take me out to dinner to thank me. Two of them said I should write it up in an article," he said. "The nice thing is, both herbs have a modest aphrodisiac effect, whereas Proscar (the most common prescription drug for prostate trouble) can cause impotence and loss of libido. Saw palmetto and pygeum do not."

Favorite Combination

Dr. Sandberg-Lewis, a faculty member and clinician at the National College of Naturopathic Medicine in Portland, recounted a couple of his cases involving saw palmetto and pygeum.

One middle-aged gentleman, recently married to a rather younger woman, lamented his complete loss of libido because of the Proscar he was taking for benign prostatic hyperplasia (BPH). He wanted to discontinue Proscar, but his medical doctor told him the only option was surgery: pulling out bits of the prostate through the urethra to alleviate the pressure on his urinary tract. That sounded pretty unappealing to this patient, so he consulted Dr. Sandberg-Lewis, who prescribed a combination of saw palmetto and pygeum. The herbs worked just as well as Proscar for preventing the urinary symptoms of BPH, while increasing his libido and enhancing his performance—definitely what the doctor ordered for this newlywed.

Dr. Sandberg-Lewis recalled another patient whose case demonstrates the effect of what we eat and drink on prostate health. When the saw palmetto—pygeum combination did not abate the BPH symptoms in this patient, Dr. Sandberg-Lewis asked about his dietary habits. The man brewed his own beer at home and, of course, sampled his product frequently. As we shall see at the end of this chapter, beer helps trigger the chemical interaction that fools the prostate into enlarging itself. An additional culprit in this case was the man's daily ration of bacon. Research by Michael Murray, N.D., indicates pork products can also exacerbate prostate problems. The home-brewer found it rather hard to give up both completely, so he and his doctor worked out a compromise plan, and the herbs were able to go to work to alleviate the BPH symptoms.

Is Pygeum Right for Me?

Pygeum is a good choice for men who want to preserve their healthy prostate, or who want to address BPH symptoms. If your life is especially stressful, this particular herb offers the added benefit of helping to balance the adrenal glands' response to stress by moderating the release of hormones like adrenaline. As we mentioned in the first chapter, The Right Chemistry, adrenal health is crucial for keeping yourself on an even keel and being able to bounce back from stress.

FLOWER POLLEN

Pollen is produced by most plants. Some of the most common pollens used to promote the health of men's urinary tracts are timothy grass, corn, rye, and pine. We don't really know why those particular plants became the most widely used, and it may be that other plant pollens are beneficial to men's health, too.

Ancient Roots

I haven't uncovered any ancient uses of flower pollen. It has been used for BPH symptoms in Europe for about 40 years.

How It Works

If you're suffering the symptoms of BPH, it's amazing how the need to urinate comes to dominate your existence. The active components of the flower pollen extract have been shown to help in two ways:

• Anti-inflammatory action helps the bladder contract and expel urine.

• Relaxation of the urethra allows easy passage of urine.

Not having to worry about these simple functions will allow you to keep your attention riveted on your partner in your intimate moments.

Research: Sexy Results

Study after study shows pollen is effective in reducing symptoms of benign prostatic hyperplasia, and as we have described previously, a healthy prostate is vital to a healthy sex life.

Several double blind studies have demonstrated that, on average, flower pollen is very effective in relieving BPH symptoms in more than 70 percent of men who use it. Among the many journals that have reported the findings on flower pollen are the highly respected *British Journal of Urology* and *Prostate*. Dr. R. Yasumoto and his associates, as reported in the *Journal of Clinical Therapeutics* in 1995, found that 85 percent of men experienced reduced BPH symptoms after taking flower pollen.

From my experience, I believe the level of success can be even higher when prostate symptoms are caught early. I think the reason those numbers are not higher is that most of the research on BPH is with men 50 and older. For example, in Yasumoto's study, the average age of the men who participated in the study was 68. I bring up the age issue because, due to the way the studies are designed, it is easy to dismiss BPH as an old man's problem. The sad part of it is these men probably experienced the classic urination symptoms of BPH for many years before they felt the need to seek medical attention. That means they may have experienced, unnecessarily, diminished sexual ability and desire for decades, thinking them the necessary corollary of aging. If you pay attention to those symptoms I listed at the beginning of this chapter and begin taking herbal remedies when you notice them, you may be one of those lucky men who enjoy sexual vigor well into their 80s and beyond.

Side Effects

There are no known side effects. Some clinicians have postulated that if a person has severe hayfever, this product may contribute to allergy symptoms. However, I have not seen this in my practice, nor have any of my colleagues.

Not for Everyone

There are no known negative interactions of flower pollen with other herbal or pharmacological medicines.

The Formula That Works

The brand of standardized flower pollen that has been most researched is Cernilton, and it is readily available throughout Europe and the United States. The dosage is 60–120 mg, 3 times a day.

Is Pollen Right for Me?

This is just one more tool in your arsenal against BPH symptoms. If for some reason another herb hasn't worked for you, pollen presents another option.

STINGING NETTLES

Stinging nettles, also known as *Urtica dioica*, contain some of the same ingredients as muira puama and pygeum for preventing and reversing BHP, alleviating the sexual problems that accompany this condition. This hardy plant can be seen on nature walks throughout temperate regions around the world. Though it presents a pretty and delicate array of greenish-white flowers, don't be drawn too close—nettles can give a nasty sting to those who brush against the hairs and bristles on the plant. The stinging comes from the presence on the bristles of chemicals such as histamine, which is also the chemical in our body that causes all those dreaded allergy symptoms, inflammation, and nasal congestion.

Ancient roots

Stinging nettles have been commonly used by Native Americans to increase urinary flow and lessen residual urine volume in the bladder. It has been used to help alleviate the symptoms of prostatitis and swelling of the prostate associated with benign prostate hyperplasia (BPH). The flowering plant and root are the medicinal parts.

How Stinging Nettles Work

For purposes of men's sexual health, the key ingredients in stinging nettles are the sterols, those hormonal building blocks, beta sitosterol, stigmasterol, campesterol, and others, which we also find in saw palmetto and pygeum. The sterols appear to lessen the action of dihydrotestosterone (DHT), the form of testosterone that causes the prostate to trick itself into creating more cells and enlarging itself, as I described in the section on saw palmetto. By preventing or minimizing prostate enlargement, you reduce the pressure on structures around the prostate and allow all the equipment to function at peak potential, whether in the bedroom or the bathroom.

As we have seen, each herb discussed in this chapter offers some similar benefits, while each has its own special bonuses. In this case, the bonus is that stinging nettles contain serotonin, one of several neurotransmitters in the brain and the main target for most anti-depressants, which increase serotonin levels to elevate mood. Acetylcholine, a neurotransmitter that targets memory, is also present. Stinging nettles also contain immune-stimulating chemicals in common with herbs such as echinacea.

Research: Sexy Results

Several researchers have shown that stinging nettles block the binding of free-floating testosterone with a protein called human sex hormone–binding globulin (SHBG). Stinging nettles can keep your testosterone circulating freely and keep you feeling sexually vital.

Side Effects

The only reported interaction is that stinging nettles may intensify the anti-inflammatory effects of diclofenac, a nonsteroidal anti-inflammatory drug (NSAID) used as a pain-reliever, similar to ibuprofen, naproxen, and aspirin. This can result in some gastrointestinal discomfort.

Not for Everyone

There are no known conditions that contraindicate men taking this herb. There is some evidence that freeze-dried nettles may increase the likelihood of miscarriage and bleeding, so pregnant women should use avoid using this botanical remedy.

The Formula That Works

For some reason we don't quite understand, the form of stinging nettles that works the best is freeze-dried; I recommend taking capsules or tablets of 300–500 mg, 3–4 times a day. This herb is also available as a tea, which you can brew by using one tablespoon of herb per 8 ounces of water, taken 3–4 times a day. Or you can try the alcohol-based tincture, administered via a dropper, at a dosage of 30 drops, 3–4 times a day. I have to warn you though, tinctures generally taste terrible because they are so highly concentrated. If you have very sensitive taste buds, you may want to choose the capsules.

The German E Commission's recommended dosage of the raw herb is 4–6 grams daily.

Are Stinging Nettles Right for Me?

As we have seen in this chapter, many of these herbs have similar benefits to the prostate and men's health in general, so to help you decide whether stinging nettles are right for you, check this list of conditions. If you experience any of these, you are likely to receive multiple benefits from stinging nettles beyond its positive effect on your prostate and your sex life:

- Hayfever
- Sinusitus
- Asthma
- Eczema

MORE THAN HERBS

A good doctor looks at the big picture, and there is more to men's sexual health than these herbs, important as they are. I've added a few basic tips you may want to consider for the long run to maintain your sexual vitality.

Zinc for Sex

Zinc is by far the most important mineral for male sexual health. Adequate zinc is critical for testosterone production, sperm formation, and prostate health. The tip-off is that the male sexual tract has the highest concentrations of zinc in the body. Zinc supplements help ensure overall virility, whether it be sexual functioning or sperm formation. Foods rich in zinc include seeds and nuts, which also offer essential fatty acids demonstrated to help maintain prostate health. In this area, science has validated another folk remedy. It has long been believed that consuming a quarter cup of pumpkin seeds once a day can lessen prostate symptoms. Since pumpkin seeds are rich in both zinc and essential fatty acids, it looks like the folk healers were right again.

Can the Beer

Sorry, guys, but beer has been strongly linked to BPH. A 17-year study in Hawaii of more than 6500 men showed that consuming 25 ounces or more of alcohol (that's only three bottles of beer!) a month was directly correlated with prostate enlargement. Beer causes a rise in the levels of prolactin, a hormone made in the pituitary gland. A rise in prolactin can cause an artificial increase in testosterone, which leads to increased creation of DHT, the culprit that causes the enlargement of the prostate. Both zinc and vitamin B6 can help reduce prolactin levels, but don't use that as an excuse to keep drinking. These nutrients may, however, offset some of the long-term effects of previous beer guzzling.

Lower cholesterol

Sexual health presents yet another reason to control cholesterol levels. Metabolic byproducts of cholesterol can accumulate in the prostate and increase the chance of prostate enlargement and even prostate cancer. BPH symptoms generally improve when cholesterol levels drop. As a bonus, lower cholesterol levels help ensure that your circulatory system is ready to perform at the drop of a hat—or anything else.

Eat These Foods

Eating a diet high in protein can inhibit the enzyme (5-alpha reductase) that converts testosterone into damaging DHT. In contrast, a diet high in carbohydrates actually stimulates production of DHT. One study found that a diet consisting of 45% protein, 35% complex carbohydrates, and 20% fat (mostly unsaturated) was effective in reducing accumulation of DHT. While this high protein level is not recommended for those with kidney problems, it could be beneficial for men under a doctor's care to reduce DHT. Also, eat lots of raw nuts and seeds, since they are naturally high in zinc and healthful fatty acids.

Avoid These Foods

Fried foods and excess red meat can lead to increased inflammation, hardening of the arteries, and reduced blood supply to the penis by causing temporary constriction of blood vessels. Also, much of the meat available in the U.S. contains myriad hormones, injected or fed to animals to increase yield, that can contribute to an imbalance of your own hormones. For the best performance in the bedroom, cut down on these foods at the table.

Let's move on to another absorbing interest of men—what gets women hot.

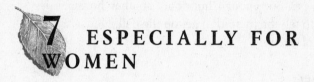

7 ESPECIALLY FOR WOMEN

As we saw in Chapter 6, Especially for Men, some herbs have gender-specific benefits that help to keep the sexual equipment in good working order. In this chapter, we will turn our attention to herbs that offer parallel benefits for women's sexual health.

When we examine natural substances that are used frequently to nourish a woman's sexual vitality, we are basically referring to herbs that help regulate female hormone levels and create an optimal balance. Hormones such as estrogen, progesterone, cortisol (released in response to stress), and testosterone all play a critical role in your sex life and overall sense of well being. Too much estrogen and you're moody; too little progesterone and you've got premenstrual symptoms that won't quit. An imbalance between these two can make you feel bloated and achy. If you are under prolonged stress, cortisol puts a damper on your sex drive. Let's take a look at this chapter's hormonal players that set the scene for your romantic encounters and see where they come from, what they do, and how an upset in their balance can affect your sex life.

Hormones Galore

We are constantly awash in a sea of hormones, secreted by various organs that act like quality-control officers to ensure your metabolism keeps running smoothly. Most hormones even have back-up hormones, such as the thyroid; if it doesn't put out enough hormone, another hormone is triggered to tell the thyroid to get on the ball. Here are just a few key players:

Estrogen.

Estrogen is a woman's primary sex hormone. It is secreted by the ovaries and determines sexual characteristics such as roundness of breast, hips, and thighs; silkiness of hair and skin; and of course, sexual preparedness, such as lubrication and health of the vagina. An estrogen deficiency can result in thinning of vaginal tissue (referred to medically as atrophic vaginitis), which can make sex uncomfortable. An excess of estrogen can result in premenstrual symptoms such as weight gain and mood swings. Too much estrogen also frequently leads to heavy menstruation that can cause anemia and fatigue, which is likely to drain you of sexual desire, as well.

Testosterone.

Every woman has a little testosterone secreted by the adrenal glands in the form of androgen. This hormone plays comparable, if lesser, roles in women as it does in men: It fuels the sex drive, contributes to physical endurance and muscle mass, and helps ward off depression.

Progesterone.

Progesterone is also a principal sex hormone for women, secreted by the ovaries. It governs the health of the uterine lining, keeping all in readiness for the arrival of a fertilized egg, and helps make sure that a pregnancy is successful. It seldom occurs that a woman produces too much progesterone; the most likely scenario is too little. This leads to extended, sometimes unremitting, menstruation, weight gain in the hips and thighs, and often premenstrual symptoms that make you want to jump out of your skin.

Prolactin.

Secreted by the pituitary gland, prolactin is the hormone responsible for increase in breast size during and after pregnancy, and triggers the formulation of breast milk. Elevated prolactin levels lead to overall PMS symptoms, and especially those pertaining to breast pain. Fibrocystic breast disease has also been attributed to increased prolactin levels.

Cortisol.

Cortisol is a hormone released by the adrenal glands in response to stress, among other things. We talked in Chapter 1: The Right Chemistry, about the need for being relaxed for better sex. If your body has been flooded by cortisol because of a stressful incident at work, for example, your system feels the effects for hours afterward. You won't feel very romantic. Instead, you'll be edgy and wonder why you haven't unwound even though you've been at home a while. If you are under prolonged stress, you'll be harder to live with—and to love. The effects of long-term stress include a shorter temper, more frequent outbursts, and difficulty getting out of bed in the morning. While cortisol imbalance affects men as well as women, there are some gender-specific results that can affect a woman's sex life negatively, namely thinning of the vaginal walls, which can make sex distinctly unpleasurable.

Thyroid.

Aside from your sex- and stress-related hormones, there's another player that serves in a crucial role: the thyroid. This small, butterfly-shaped gland at the base of your throat secretes thyroxine, which determines not only how well your sex-related hormones work, but the general efficiency of your entire metabolism. In fact, if your thyroid is out of balance, secreting too much or too little thyroxine, nothing—and I mean *nothing*—will be able to function optimally.

Check yourself for these common symptoms of abnormal thyroid function. With hypothyroidism (low thyroxine), you may experience symptoms such as weight gain with no meaningful change in diet, slower thinking, slower bowels, sense of being cold (frequently associated with lower body temperature), and, often, substantially decreased libido. With hyperthyroidism (high thyroxine), you may experience symptoms such as mood swings, anxiety, weight loss, sweating, irregular menstruation, insomnia, and a swelling at the base of your throat. If you experience any of these symptoms, visit your doctor. A simple blood test can offer you peace of mind.

A Healthy Balance

The balancing act of our many hormones is critical to our general sense of well-being, including our readiness for sex. While the male hormone testosterone governs a woman's sex drive, it is important to remember that the female hormones determine a woman's ability to respond to her sex drive. Hormones like estrogen and progesterone influence physical responsiveness that contributes hugely to sexual pleasure and desire, such as vaginal lubrication; excitability of vulva, clitoris, and vaginal tissues; mood; and general readiness for a sexual rendezvous. But see what happens to your sex life if your hormonal balance is off-kilter.

For example, if estrogen and progesterone levels are out of balance (most commonly high estrogen, low progesterone), you may experience symptoms such as fluid retention, bloating, breast tenderness, lack of lubrication, decreased sexual desire, mood swings, and depression. Other hormonal imbalance symptoms include those oft-cited headaches, thinning of vaginal walls, and frequent urinary tract infections, not to mention forgetfulness, lack of mental clarity, and cold hands and feet. An unseen symptom is depressed liver function, and since this organ is responsible for filtering out waste chemicals, that means it will have a harder time ridding the system of the excess estrogen! There are some other physical symptoms that can indicate if you have an imbalance of these two hormones, such as changes in the texture of your skin or hair, an unexplained weight gain, or changes in breast or hip size unrelated to body weight.

The herbs we will discuss in this chapter are known specifically for their ability to balance hormonal levels and nourish a woman's overall wellness. For instance, dong quai has an ancient reputation as such an effective herb for women that it is called the "female ginseng." Wild yam has many supporters and some detractors, but it is very popular among herbalists. Cimicifuga (black cohosh) was used by Native Americans and others to support women's sexual functions. Using herbs like these to improve your hormonal balance can make the difference between whether the testosterone spark of your sexual urge will ignite passion, or fizzle out. Of course, it is possible to have sex when you're feeling less than your best, and some people say there's no such thing as bad sex. But when you're aiming for great sex, you want to achieve that hormonal balance to feel really in the groove. Here are some herbs that can help you get there.

DONG QUAI

Although this herb grows indigenously around the world, it is most widely known by its Chinese name, dong quai (in other dialects, dang gui or tang-kuei). The Latin botanical name for this plant is *Angelica sinensis*. It is one of numerous *angelica* species; European varieties include *Angelica officinalis* or *Angelica archangelica*; the American variety is *Angelica atropurpurea*.

Dong quai boasts beautiful greenish-white flowers beginning in May and lasting throughout the summer. The delicate flowers present themselves in a semi-circle, or umbrella, shape. The serrated leaves form a lacy backdrop to the bloom, and the sturdy stalk is slightly furrowed on the outside and mostly hollow on the inside. Species such as *Angelica archangelica* can grow to a height of seven feet. This herb prefers habitats that are damp and cool, such as meadows, coastal regions, mountainous areas, and along rivers. In Asia, dong quai is cultivated for medicinal applications, whereas in modern Europe and the United States, it is used more frequently as a flavoring for such foods as ice cream, candy, vermouths, puddings, gelatins, and beverages. It also flavors the liqueurs Chartreuse and Benedictine, and is added to juniper berries to make gin.

Regardless of the species *angelica*, all varieties share membership in the celery family, a delightful reminder that our food and our medicine are not so separate as modern science would have them seem.

Ancient Roots

In both Europe and Asia, *angelica* has a historical track record of medicinal use. In China, where dong quai has been used for more than 2,000 years, it is called the "female ginseng" because of its tonic effects on women's reproductive system. Historically, it has been prescribed for uterine bleeding, painful menses, scant menstrual flow, and abnormal menstrual cycle. After menopause, dong quai is administered to ease symptoms such as hot flashes, night sweats, and mood swings. This herb is also used for high blood pressure and poor circulation in the hands and feet. Traditionally, the parts of the plant used are the root and lower part of the stem, called the rhizome.

In medieval Europe, gardeners in Norway, Iceland, and Greenland grew angelica, and twelfth century legal texts state that a tenant farmer who had an angelica garden must be allowed to take the plants when he moved, according to Suzanne Fischer-Rizzi in *Medicine of the Earth*. She goes on to describe how, in the Fourteenth Century, monks brought the plant from these northern countries to southern Europe, and during the Middle Ages, the root was considered a kind of panacea and was believed effective against the plague and any type of contagious disease. This parallels the Chinese belief in dong quai as a blood purifier.

China's use of dong quai was so pervasive that a few centuries ago it became too scarce to export, and Japan was left to cultivate its native species, *Angelica acutiloba,* instead of importing dong quai from China. This has led each country to attach special properties to its native species, and it is now widely held by each culture that the other's *angelica* is weak and of little medicinal benefit, whereas the scientific literature actually demonstrates that both species are similarly effective.

How It Works

Dong quai is still used today by clinicians in modern practices to help relieve the same symptoms associated with the ancient use of the herb. My patients have experienced success in taking dong quai for premenstrual symptoms (including mood swings, water retention, and anxiety); it also proves helpful for painful menses. It is effective against menopausal symptoms as well, including night sweats and hot flashes. For my patients suffering from menopausal symptoms, I often will add black cohosh to my recommendations because of the synergy between the two herbs, which I will discuss further in the section on black cohosh. Most patients using dong quai report feeling "better in their skin," that is, more balanced, with greater clarity, inner energy, and a generally improved sense of well being.

Dong quai contains many nutrients, from metals like cobalt, copper, and manganese, to plant sterols, which have similar chemical structures, to hormones like estrogen, progesterone, and testosterone, and like the beta sitosterol in saw palmetto. It also has more readily recognizable elements like calcium, potassium, vitamins E and B-12, and pantothenic acid. Among the ingredients with active medicinal properties are coumarins (which can help optimize a woman's overall health), essential oils, and various flavonoids.

Though the plant sterols in dong quai are not nearly as strong as animal-based estrogen, they pack enough power to give dong quai a dual effect: The herb lowers excess estrogen activity in some women, while stimulating estrogen activity in those who need it, resulting in a balance for both cases. Here's how it works. The cells in a woman's body that are designed to respond to estrogen, such as those in the vagina and breast, have what are called estrogen receptors that recognize the action of this hormone. In a woman with excess estrogen (demonstrated by weight gain, mood swings, and other premenstrual symptoms that won't quit), dong quai's plant sterols, weakly mimicking estrogen, trigger competition among estrogen receptors, resulting in a dilution of the estrogen effect. In a woman with low estrogen, dong quai combines with the woman's naturally occurring hormonal levels to activate estrogen receptors that otherwise might not be stimulated. As we discussed earlier in this chapter, proper estrogen levels are required to enhance a woman's responsiveness to sexual overtures. Also, modulating the estrogen activity is important because high estrogen can be a contributing factor to breast and colon cancer.

As mentioned earlier, dong quai also has been prescribed through the ages for painful menses, and now we know that the herb has painkilling properties measured at 1.7 times the effect of aspirin. Also, the essential oils present in dong quai have antispasmodic properties to relax smooth muscles, which reinforces the historical use of this herb for menstrual cramps. These properties may also be applied to other painful conditions such as headaches and arthritis, but these uses require further studies to better document dong quai's medicinal effects.

Research: Sexy Results

Dong quai's ability to optimize female hormones sets the stage for responsiveness to sexual desire. Sexual pleasure, particularly orgasmic intensity, may be enhanced with the use of dong quai. Among the dozens of Asian studies on dong quai in the past two decades, some have shown that the Japanese species actually causes an alternating uterine contraction followed by relaxation. Many experts believe that uterine contractions during sex contribute to the height of pleasure achieved.

The dong quai species of *angelica* also confers the added benefit of antibacterial properties, possibly lessening the chance of minor infections that might affect one's sex life. However, its effects are not sufficient to actually treat an infection; rather it more likely offers a small insurance policy against conditions such as mild bladder infections and vaginal infections.

Side Effects

Like ginseng, the vast majority of women can take this herb for long periods of time with little risk of negative interaction or side effect.

Not for Everyone

Since dong quai affects hormonal balance, it is not indicated for pregnant or lactating women. Also, some fair-skinned individuals report becoming more sensitive to sunlight, so if you take dong quai and are prone to sunburn or spend a lot of time in the sun, you might consider a lotion with a higher sun protection factor (SPF). After all, few people feel very sexy when they've been broiled like a lobster!

The Formula That Works

Dong quai isn't typically standardized, but when you are selecting a brand, be sure to look for organic and/or wild-crafted plant material that hasn't been fumigated (which is often the case with imported products). This herb comes in a variety of forms and you can select the one that works best for your lifestyle.

Capsules/Tablets:
   1000 mg, 3–4 times a day

Tinctures:
   45–60 drops, 2–3 times a day

Tea:
   1 tablespoon per cup of hot water, 3–4 times a day

Is Dong Quai Right for Me?

What I have observed throughout my clinical experience is that if a given herb's therapeutic range of applications harmonizes with a patient's specific condition, then often its overall benefits are that much more substantial. This amazing herb may put a spark in your sex life regardless of whether you may have a hint or more of the following conditions:

- Allergies
- Fibrocystic breast disease
- High blood pressure
- Menopause
- Menstrual cramps
- PMS
- Poor circulation

WILD YAM

This herb grows as a perennial vine that presents small greenish yellow flowers. The root is the medicinal component. Wild yam grows in southern regions of Canada and in the United States. It grows best in the temperate, subtropical, and tropical climates. Among its more tropical habitats include South America, Mexico, and Asia. There is some confusion of terminology among herbalists between wild yam and Mexican yam, which was tapped for its estrogen precursors to create the early birth control pills. We will go with the prevailing terminology and refer to *Dioscorea villosa* as wild yam.

Ancient Roots

Although *dioscorea villosa* has a colorful past of medicinal use, I couldn't locate any historical examples of the way it was used to enhance sexual function. The medicinal components of *d. villosa* include the dried rhizome (bottom part of stem) and root. This herb has other folk names, such as Devil's bones, Yuma, Colic Root, and Rheumatism Root. Throughout the ages, it has been used for coughs, stomach and intestinal irritation, and nerve pain.

According to *Herbal Medicine Past and Present* (Duke University Press, 1990), wild yam began gaining momentum for its medicinal use in this country in the early 1800s, after John Riddell's *Synopsis of the Flora of the Western States* (1835) described *d. villosa* as "unquestionably a valuable remedy in bilious colic." It continued to gather fans throughout the century, being cited in R.E. Griffith's *Medical Botany* (1847) for its action to induce sweating and as an expectorant, and in C. H. Leonard's *Materia Medica and Therapeutics* (1891) for use against rheumatism. But the 1930 edition of the *Dispensatory of the United States* bluntly stated that it is improbable that yam possesses any real therapeutic virtues and that its infrequent use scarcely justifies official recognition.

How It Works

Only decades after this dismissive entry in the *Dispensatory of the United States,* research found that wild yam does indeed contain medicinal properties, although some of them need some pharmaceutical help to become useful. For example, yam contains the plant steroid diosgenin, which can be processed chemically into corticosteroid, widely used as an anti-inflammatory medication against joint pain, such as arthritis. What takes place in the lab, however, cannot be duplicated in the human body, so this is a good example of why a plant substance gets synthesized into a drug. However, the large amount of wild yam's diosgenin, a precursor in the chemical synthesis of progesterone, has been touted as a building block to help increase progesterone activity in a woman with a deficiency of this hormone. As mentioned earlier, progesterone has numerous functions, including uterine health and warding off symptoms of premenstrual syndrome.

In a lovely display of herbal diversity, wild yam also contains beta carotene, an antioxidant that protects against

cancer, lowers blood triglycerides, and raises HDL cholesterol (the "good" cholesterol). In addition, yam has antispasmodic and anti-inflammatory properties. This affords
practitioners and herbalists clinical use of this plant for
myriad conditions, including: inflammation, spasms (especially menstrual cramps), muscle pain, high blood lipids
(cholesterol and triglycerides), digestive problems like
diverticulitis (it increases the flow of bile from the gallbladder to help digestion, especially fat), and arthritis.

Research: Sexy Results

Research is still very sketchy on the effectiveness of this
herb. It is commonly found in numerous herbal blends and
supplements as a nutritive herb. I and other clinicians find it
helpful to patients, but it appears that its medicinal properties haven't been fully discovered by botanical researchers.
Clinically, it appears to support healthy menstrual cycles
and, specifically, lessen painful menses and cramps. Its ability to enhance sexuality is suggested, at this point in our
knowledge, by its ability to lessen menstrual disturbances,
thereby indirectly affecting an overall sense of wellness.

Side Effects

There are very few side effects associated with this herb. It
is generally considered safe. However, the large amount of
wild yam's diosgenin can be used by the body to support and
enhance progesterone activity in a woman with a deficiency
of this hormone. As mentioned earlier, progesterone contributes to uterine health and wards off symptoms of premenstrual syndrome.

Not for Everyone

Because of the herb's effect on hormones, this is not recommended for women who are pregnant or nursing.

The Formula That Works

Wild yam is almost always used in combination with other herbs such as angelica, black or blue cohosh, licorice, or cramp bark, that nourish women's sex-related functions. However, capsules and tablets are available, and you could safely take 500–1000 mg, 3 times a day.

Is Wild Yam Right for Me?

The benefits of wild yam are more nutritive and less directly hormonal, and I believe that it is fine for you to try a moderate dose if you have some of the menstrual difficulties we describe in this chapter. The real key when taking herbs is to listen to your body. If symptoms don't improve or a new symptom appears, I always recommend discontinuing.

BLACK COHOSH

This shrublike plant grows throughout forested areas in eastern North America. It can be found as far south as Georgia, as far west as Arkansas, and as far north as Ontario. The plant sprouts to a height of 3–4 feet. Its medicinal roots are straight and a dark brownish color. Though it grows indigenously in the U.S. and parts of Canada, it is also cultivated in Europe.

Ancient Roots

Black cohosh is also known in Latin as *Cimicifuga racemosa*. The term "cohosh" was used by Native Americans to describe the rough appearance of the roots, which were harvested for medicinal purposes. They can be used either fresh or dried. Prior to European colonization of America, natives used it for everything from rattlesnake bites to various women's health issues. During the mid-1800s, American physicians prescribed black cohosh for conditions such as arthritis, insomnia, menstrual cramps, and symptoms of influenza. Other common names that are frequently used for this herb include: rattleweed, rattleroot, black snake root, richweed, bugwort, and squaw root.

How It Works

Black cohosh contains numerous chemical constituents. Among the components that are believed to possess medicinal properties are isoflavones, like formononetin, which mimic hormonal activity. Laboratory studies show that formononetin, when taken orally, can bind onto estrogen receptors, which supports the possibility that this herb may have some hormonal regulation properties. Yet sufficient studies still need to occur before conclusive clinical results can be drawn.

That said, black cohosh has been used for more than 40 years throughout most of Europe with outstanding success. There is a growing body of evidence to suggest that this humble-looking yet dynamic herb delivers a powerful hormonal punch. Here's how it works: Your pituitary gland secretes luteinizing hormone (LH) and follicle stimulating hormone (FSH) to keep your estrogen and progesterone production in the right balance. High LH and FSH levels usually mean your estrogen and progesterone production and balance are out of kilter. In studies conducted in Germany, researchers E.M. Duker and his colleagues found that when the women in the study took black cohosh, LH and FSH levels decreased, suggesting that this herb influences production and balance of estrogen and progesterone to maintain the health of the uterus and vagina.

Research: Sexy Results

In the study mentioned above, reported in *Plant Medicine* (1991), 110 menopausal women were treated with an alcohol extract of black cohosh (Remifemin®) at a dose of 8 milligrams per day, or a placebo. Eight weeks later, LH levels were decreased in the women who took the black cohosh. These results suggest an estrogenic effect. Increased estrogen can enhance your sense of sexual receptiveness, help with vaginal lubrication, and make you feel more vital and healthy.

Side Effects

Since it has the ability to alter hormonal balance, black cohosh should be avoided by women who are either pregnant or lactating. Among possible side effects, though not particularly common, are: stomach discomfort, headache, dizziness, and nausea. Women using pharmaceutical estrogen replacement should not take black cohosh without a health care practitioner's guidance, since there can be a synergistic effect that can lead to signs and symptoms of excessive estrogen levels. At very high doses, low blood pressure and limb pain might occur. The most common side effect that one might experience, if sensitive, is stomach upset.

Not For Everyone

Black cohosh should not be used by women who are pregnant, due to its ability to cause bleeding. It may result in breakthrough bleeding and miscarriage. Black cohosh should also not be used by lactating women because of the potential of toxicity for the child.

The Formula That Works

When you are selecting a brand of black cohosh, be sure to look for organic or wildcrafted and standardized, if available, in a base of whole herb. This herb comes in a variety of forms and you can select the one that works best for your lifestyle.

Dried unprocessed root:
    500 mg, 2–4 times a day

Tablets/capsules:
    500 mg, 1–2 times a day (powdered)

Standardized tablets:
    2 times a day (depending on dosage) 2 mg of 27-deoxy-actecine—an indicator of the strength of the extract)

Tincture:
    1 teaspoon, 2–3 times a day

As I mentioned earlier, I often recommend a combination formula of black cohosh with dong quai because the two have complementary effects that benefit many women who suffer symptoms of PMS or menopause. Dong quai's tonic effect can increase energy and improve mood while black cohosh goes to work to redress the imbalance of estrogen and progesterone that gives rise to symptoms like sweating, bloating, and abdominal discomfort that make a woman feel drained or out of sorts. In Appendix A, I will talk about proportions and amounts of herbs that are most effective in combination.

Is Black Cohosh Right for Me?

If you suffer from menopausal symptoms, menstrual pain, or uterine spasm, you are likely to benefit from black cohosh. This herb also helps women who experience mood swings or feel out of sorts or spacy during menstruation. Many of my female patients find black cohosh to be an excellent remedy time and again. This amazing herb also helps those who have entered natural or surgically induced menopause with similar symptoms. I have also seen black cohosh help anxiety that stems from hormonal fluctuations and help mild depression that can result from monthly hormonal cycles.

Before we move on, I want to say a brief word about the hormonal action of the herbs we discuss in this chapter. In my opinion, it is potentially dangerous to self-prescribe hormones, whether they be progesterone or other popular hormones like DHEA or melatonin. Some herbs can have powerful hormonal effects, and I believe balancing your hormones is a matter that requires consultation with your healthcare provider.

MORE THAN HERBS

Herbs can make a valuable contribution to a vibrant sex life, but they cannot overcome the cumulative effects of poor lifestyle choices. We will cover these choices more extensively in a later chapter, but here are some tips especially for women to help preserve not only physical charms but inner balance and overall health.

Exercise

You've heard it a hundred times from dozens of sources, because it's true: Exercise is important to maintain overall health. Many of us get tired of hearing the "e" word because it always sounds like work, but it doesn't have to be. Let's call it doing something fun: any activity such as biking, gardening, skiing of any kind, horseback riding, dancing, hiking, strolling around the park, and, yes, sex! Although it is difficult for some of us to manage the really active part of sex (that can last for 20–30 minutes, long enough to get the heart rate to climb), the herbs we discuss in this book will surely help you increase your stamina!

What I'm telling you is, anything that gets you out of that chair is a good thing. Here's what activity will do for you:

You sweat, which is good for your skin—you get rid of toxins, your skin glows, and those tiny facial lines you slather with lotion will be hydrated naturally. Also, studies show that menopausal women who are active on a regular basis (3.5 hours a week) have fewer and less intense hot flashes than women who don't. One study found that *all* the active women could skip hormone replacement therapy. Take care of your body, and it takes care of you! Women who are active also have a better outlook on life and score higher mood ratings on tests, a wonderful example of the mind-body connection.

Smoking

Again, I know you've heard it before, but smoking poses gender-specific risks to women. It actually seems to upset the hormonal balance, according to research that shows women who smoke have twice the risk of starting menopause early. It has also been shown that the early onset of menopause may be reversed to some degree, upon cessation of smoking. The longer you menstruate, the longer you are producing your own estrogen, which keeps you looking youthful. Smoking puts you at risk of ending your natural cycle prematurely, and while your estrogen production will slow down eventually, smoking invites it to occur early, which you want to avoid.

Foods for Balance

Research is starting to suggest that certain foods have pro-hormonal effects that can lessen mood swings and help modulate the symptoms of minor hormonal imbalance. The most important is soy. An interesting fact is that one cup of soybeans yields 300 milligrams of isoflavones, chemicals that seem to help balance the body's systems, like the tonifying herbs ginseng and ashwagandha, that improve the body's general function. Soy is one reason why Asians who adhere to their traditional diet have a much lower incidence of cancer.

One easy way to get soy into your diet is to substitute tofu (soybean curd) for chicken in your next stir-fry. Tofu takes on any flavor and can be stir-fried or baked into many dishes. Although this typically Asian staple is now readily available in grocery stores, Americans seem to have a tough time buying a block of "gelatinous white stuff." But soy is so nutritious and inexpensive that food manufacturers are going out of their way to make it a little more visually appealing. They now disguise it as cold cuts, sliced cheese, and what one patient of mine calls "faux" (false) meat that looks like ground hamburger or breakfast sausage. Roasted soybeans make a tasty, crunchy snack, too.

Other important foods suspected of having hormonal effects include celery, fennel, parsley, and various nuts and seeds. Flaxseed oil and fiber are high in lignans, which have the same hormone-mimicking quality of soy's isoflavones and are also popularly used by nutritionally oriented physicians.

Essential Fatty Acids

Given all the negative publicity that fat has received, it's hard to believe that some fats are very important to have in your diet. These are called "essential fatty acids," EFA for short. It has been estimated that only 1 in 6 Americans get enough EFAs. A very common sign of essential fatty acid deficiency is little "goose bump"-like spots on the back of your arms and possibly elsewhere that don't go away. In women, EFA deficiency can aggravate any tendency toward menstrual cramps.

This is easily remedied by taking a tablespoon of flaxseed oil per day (straight or in juices, smoothies, or even on salad). You can also find capsules of EFA, but they are more expensive than the oil. Even more economical is to buy bulk flaxseeds at your local health-food store and incorporate them into salads, breads, cereals, or nut butters. One of my women patients read the label of the flaxseed oil bottle and said, "You want me to add 10 grams of fat to my diet on purpose? Are you nuts?" The benefits are well worth the few calories. It will help you get rid of dry skin, lessen or eliminate those annoying little bumps, and provide a more silky looking complexion. Correcting an EFA deficiency can also lessen muscle and joint pain and help with mental clarity. Essential fatty acids can make you feel good—and look good—and this, of course, also helps to revitalize your sex life.

Magnesium

Do you crave chocolate? Maybe this is really your body's way of telling you it needs magnesium. Women who crave chocolate often have this deficiency and chocolate is certainly a pleasant way to supply it. Of course, you know the downside of too much self-medicating with chocolate (weight gain, for one), but pay attention to that magnesium deficiency. Magnesium is a crucial ingredient to energy production in the cells. Without sufficient magnesium, your body can't produce energy efficiently, and this will certainly impact your interest in and ability to respond to sexual invitations.

Rice Bran Oil

Also known as ferulic acid or gamma oryzanol, rice bran oil is considered a tissue builder. It has been widely used to heal wounds, lower cholesterol, and relieve the symptoms of hormonal imbalance such as premenstrual symptoms. Rice bran oil is also effective against menopausal symptoms. You can find this in most health-food stores. A typical dose would be 50–100 mg, 3 times a day.

Vitamin C with Bioflavonoids

Vitamin C helps the body make strong and resilient collagen. Most of you are aware that collagen helps you have that fresh, youthful complexion and touchable looking skin all over. To get the best effect of vitamin C, I usually recommend taking it in a base of bioflavonoids, chemicals that occur naturally with vitamin C in foods such as oranges or grapefruits, because this combination increases the vitamin's absorption and activity by about 35 percent. If the vitamin C content is 500–1000 mg, the bioflavonoid content should be 50–100 mg; or you can take a popular combination of vitamin C with rose hips, which is a natural source of balanced vitamin C and bioflavonoids. Such combinations also improve circulation and may prevent or lessen the occurrence of varicose or spider veins. Long-term use is recommended to achieve these benefits.

Vitamin E

Though I don't recommend that you self-prescribe vitamin E in vaginal suppository form, I have had great success with it. Use of the suppositories can markedly improve the health of vaginal tissue in ways such as relieving vaginal dryness or reversing the thinning of tissues. The mechanism for this may have been uncovered in a study that shows vitamin E increases the blood supply to vaginal tissues, and it is the blood that supplies the nutrients that keep you healthy. Vitamin E also lessens menopausal symptoms. Check with your doctor to see if this is right for you.

These are just a few suggestions especially for women, and in Chapter 10, we'll be examining some overall lifestyle issues that can hamper or help your sexual enjoyment. First, though, let's take a look at some herbs with reputations as aphrodisiacs, and see if they live up to the claim.

8 FACT OR FOLKLORE?

Many herbs have historical and cultural reputations for aphrodisiac properties. Sometimes this is justified, as we have seen in the preceding chapters, but other herbs have more folklore than fact to back up claims on their behalf. The substances we discuss in this chapter have historical reputations as aphrodisiacs, but have less scientific documentation or research supporting their claims to sexual enhancement than those we have already addressed. As we examine the evidence for each of them in the research section, we'll assess which end of the spectrum they fall on—fact or folklore—and I will rate them from a ho-hum one star to a "check this out" five stars.

In this chapter, we will travel from India to the New World to review a few ancient and well-respected herbs in the natural pharmacopeia of indigenous peoples and their reputed effects on sexual enhancement. We will also examine an amino acid found in numerous foods that is the subject of increasing scholarly research for its use in several conditions, and which is being used by some clinicians as a natural substitute for Viagra.

ASHWAGANDHA

A member of the pepper family, ashwagandha is native to India and Africa, and is a vital component of Ayurvedic medicine, the 2,500-year-old system of healing native to India. The ashwagandha shrub bears edible seeds, but the medicinal component is the root. This plant is considered a food to people in Africa and India, who use its shoots and seeds to thicken milk.

Ancient Roots

Traditional uses of *Withania somniferum,* ashwagandha's botanical name, have included treatment of tumors, inflammation, arthritis, and a variety of infectious diseases. It is also an ingredient in sex tonics. We can expect to learn much from India about what enhances sex, since this is the culture that gave the world one of its first sex manuals, the *Kama Sutra.*

How It Works

The chemically active ingredients in ashwagandha are substances called withanolides, purported to be the source of many of this plant's medicinal properties. Withanolides appear to have a steroid-like effect, meaning that they indirectly increase activity among steroidal hormones like testosterone and progesterone. Because testosterone is a star player when it comes to our sex drive, this mechanism could potentially be responsible for ashwagandha's purported aphrodisiac effect.

Withanolides also seem to have properties similar to panax (Asian) ginseng, and ashwagandha has been referred to as "Indian ginseng." Like panax ginseng, ashwagandha is revered as a non-specific tonic, an "adaptogen" that is used alone or as an ingredient in compounds designed to target a variety of conditions. As you will recall from the gingko and ginseng chapters, a tonic with adaptogenic properties is an overall "good-for-what-ails-you" medicine: It relaxes you when you feel stressed and energizes you when you feel tired.

As with gingko and ginseng, ashwagandha appears to stimulate circulation by relaxing the blood vessels, and we have discussed at length in those earlier chapters the critical role of circulation in sexual performance. Circulation gets all the chemical messages where they need to go and primes the pump to set the stage for good sexual performance.

Research: Sexy Results

Research indicates that Ashwagandha's reputation as an aphrodisiac probably stems mainly from its ability to stimulate an overall sense of wellbeing. This sounds simplistic, but when was the last time you rolled out of bed and felt utterly joyful to be alive? Sadly, a sense of wellbeing has become a goal in our lives instead of our normal state of existence.

Like panax ginseng, ashwagandha helps us withstand and prevail over the stress of our hectic lives. In one experiment, 34 people suffering from anxiety underwent a baseline test of their brain activity, and another test after being treated with ashwagandha for 12 weeks. The test results showed that their brain chemistry actually changed in that time, from activity patterns reflecting anxiety to homeostasis, the scientific term for the normal balance of our system, which is necessary for us to thrive. The study participants' experience echoed the test results: They reported a greater sense of wellness.

Researchers speculate the anti-anxiety action of ashwaganda stems from something in the herb that mimics gamma-amino-butyric acid (GABA), a chemical that occurs naturally in the brain. GABA's role is to decrease the effect of stimuli that reach the brain. Therapeutically, many antiepileptic drugs actually increase GABA levels to decrease neurological overstimulation. If you are experiencing a lot of stress, GABA can help keep you from feeling overwhelmed and prevent physical manifestations of anxiety such as the racing heart, hyperventilation, and the feeling that your heart is ready to jump out of your throat.

According to numerous European and Indian studies published by peer-reviewed journals in the past decade, ashwagandha stimulates the immune system, fights inflammation, and improves memory. (Peer-reviewed, or scholarly, journals publish only research that meets rigorous scientific standards and passes the scrutiny of experts in that particular field.) Add to this ashwagandha's effect on increased circulation and decreased anxiety levels, which research supports, and ashwagandha turns out to be just what it is purported to be: an adaptogen, an all-around "feel good" herb.

The kind of "feel-good" I am talking about is not a "buzz" kind of feeling; rather, this effect is felt in contrast. You know how stress makes you feel—tired and cranky with barely enough energy to be a couch potato. When you take ashwagandha or other adaptogens on a daily basis, after 2–4 weeks you often begin to realize you no longer feel so drained, so at the end of your rope. The stress in your life may remain the same, but the adaptogen changes the way you respond in mind and body. When this effect kicks in, you feel more energetic, more alert, more alive—and that's sexy. This is how Asians, Indians, and other ancient peoples view true aphrodisiacs: building long-term stamina, not the Western "magic bullet," pop this pill and you're ready in an hour, approach. Ashwagandha's staying power lasts much longer and, as a bonus, it promotes your overall health.

Bottom line:

With the research being conducted on ashwagandha, I'd say this adaptogen is well on its way toward moving from folklore to fact, and I give it a rating of three out of five stars.

Side Effects

A review of the research literature does not indicate any side effects of ashwagandha, nor does there appear to be any danger of toxicity. However, it is always best to start with a low dose and work up to the full amount.

Not For Everyone

The studies on ashwagandha's anti-anxiety effects lead me to recommend against taking it if you are already on any prescribed medicine for anxiety or depression. The herb may intensify a drug's action or trigger a drug's side effects. Also, ashwagandha has not been tested specifically for safe use during pregnancy and lactation, and there is some suggestion that the herb may trigger miscarriages.

The Formula That Works

Ashwagandha is available in a variety of forms. In each one of them, look for the use of the organic whole herb, standardized if available, although even the unstandardized whole herb also appears be effective. As with other herbs, expect to take this daily for 2–4 weeks before you begin to feel its beneficial effects.

- In an alcohol-based tincture, a therapeutic dosage is about 60–90 drops, 2–3 times per day.

- As a capsule or tablet, you may take 1000 mg, 1–2 times a day.

- For those who enjoy the occasional ritual and cere-
  mony of tea, you can brew a tea by boiling 1000–1500
  mg of root for 10 minutes in 16 ounces of water. You
  may take 2–3 cups of this per day.

Is Ashwagandha Right for Me?

When considering the use of ashwagandha, you'll recall
that it shares many of the tonic qualities of Chinese ginseng,
hence its popularity in India as the "Indian Ginseng." That
means it is of great benefit to those under stress who need to
call on reserves of energy and mental clarity to get through
the day and have some energy left over for a night life. If this
is your situation, you are most likely to benefit from ashwagandha. People with the following conditions are also likely
to experience this herb's benefit:

- Alzheimer's disease
- Fatigue
- HIV
- Immune deficiency
- Inflammation

SARSAPARILLA

Just imagine—sarsaparilla, the beverage of good guys in
the old West, had a reputation not only as an aphrodisiac but
as a cure for syphilis. Maybe that was the reason they served
it in saloons!

There are several varieties of this plant around the world,
but the one we are talking about is *Smilax sarsaparilla*, native
to the Southeastern United States, Mexico, Central and
South America, and throughout the Caribbean island
nations. Sarsaparilla is a perennial woody vine with prickly
stems, thick root stalks, and roots several feet long. It can
grow along the ground or climb trees, and it likes hillsides

and swamps. Sarsaparilla sports bright red berries, although its tuberous root is the medicinal component. The root has a somewhat spicy, pleasant scent and gave the original "root beer" its bite.

Ancient Roots

Like its closely related cousins in Europe and Asia, sarsaparilla has been used for centuries to treat a variety of conditions such as rheumatoid arthritis, skin ailments like eczema, infections and inflammations, and to "purify" the blood. It also has a reputation as a tonic, which, as you'll recall from the gingko and ginseng chapters, gives the system a general "tune up" to increase overall function, on the basis that the body as a whole is only as efficient and powerful as its least effective part.

The American folk herbalist Tommie Bass, whose inherited lore and decades of practice are the foundation of *Herbal Medicine Past and Present* (Duke University Press, 1990) said people native to the southeastern United States held sarsaparilla in high esteem for its blood purifying properties. "The Indians praised it to high heaven," Bass told researchers John Crellin and Jane Philpott. "They claimed it would build up an old man or an old women, or a young man or young woman. I don't think there is anything that will beat it for a blood purifier."

Sarsaparilla also has a long history of use outside its native America. In the 1500s, when a syphilis epidemic broke out in Europe, physicians believed that because the disease came from the New World, it seemed only reasonable that an herb from the New World would cure it. Sarsaparilla fitted the bill: It had a reputation as a blood purifier and it seemed effective against syphilis. For hundreds of years, the root accumulated a reputation as a cure for this and other sexually transmitted diseases. Chinese and Portuguese physicians observed that men seemed to recover more rapidly when administered sarsaparilla, and the root was registered as a syphilis treatment in the U.S. Pharmacopoeia from 1820 to 1910. By then, it had lost ground to mercury as the treatment of choice. Even though researchers now repudiate sarsaparilla's effectiveness against syphilis, it was certainly more beneficial than mercury, which killed people before the disease could!

How It Works

The exact mechanism of action for sarsaparilla has not been identified. Chemical constituents of the herb such as phytosterols, like beta sitosterol, which we also find in saw palmetto, are believed to stimulate hormone-like activity in the body. Also, research in the Twentieth Century has discovered that sarsaparilla's medicinally active ingredients include steroidal saponins, a soap-like substance. The saponins include smilasponin, sarsaparilloside, and sarsaponin, and they comprise only a tiny part of the plant's weight—less than two percent. Among the other components are aglycones (non-sugar glycogens), volatile oils (like the aromatic oils of citrus), and resins (which gave root beer its tang).

For many years, people thought sarsaparilla had testosterone in it. Though this herb has strong tonic effects, there is no testosterone present in it, or any plant studied so far. There are, however, steroid-like components: the steroidal saponins and the phytosterols that, though not readily absorbed from the digestive tract, may contribute to testosterone's activity at some level. There is conjecture among both researchers and herbalists that these steroidal compounds have anabolic activity (to increase sex drive, muscle-building) although no research yet supports this concept. Some experts in the weight training field believe that physical results in some men who use this herb, such as body building contestants, are due to increased drive and stamina, resulting from sarsaparilla's ability to fuel the energy, focus, and endurance that go into bulking up the muscles.

Research: Sexy Results

While sarsaparilla has some admirable qualities that seem to benefit overall health, I couldn't find much to substantiate any reputation as a sex tonic. That may change, since after many decades of neglect, sarsaparilla has been drawing increasing attention recently. Several scholars have studied and collected information about this tonic herb: Albert Lung and Steven Foster in their *Encyclopedia of Common Natural Ingredients*; John Heinerman in *Heinerman's Encyclopedia of Healing Herbs and Spices*; Michael Murray, N.D., in the *Healing Power of Herbs*; James A. Duke, Ph.D., in *Handbook of Medicinal Herbs*; and Daniel B. Mowrey in *Herbal Tonic Therapies*. Among the research cited in these works are studies on sarsaparilla's effectiveness as an antibiotic, an anti-inflammatory, and a treatment for leprosy and psoriasis. They even relate to that old-fashioned notion of purifying the blood, through antimicrobial action. The herb's effectiveness against psoriasis, a very stubborn skin disease, is linked to sarsaparilla's ability to lessen the absorption of toxins formed by bacteria in the intestines and its ability to decrease cholesterol reabsorption by the lower large intestine. This kind of general cleansing activity is what herbalists and holistic healers love to see, because it combats so many conditions and promotes better health.

Bottom line:

While the research indicates sarsaparilla has great potential as a system tonic, there doesn't seem to be anything indicating its use specifically for sexual function, so I give this herb two out of five stars on our scale.

Side Effects

Sarsaparilla is generally considered safe, but it has been reported that nausea and vomiting can occur when sarsaparilla is taken for a prolonged period of time. It can also interact negatively with both bismuth (popularly taken as Pepto-Bismol) and the heart medicine digitalis.

Not For Everyone

In people with kidney problems or diabetes (which can cause kidney problems), damage to the kidneys can result if sarsaparilla is taken in excessive doses (greater than 3 milliliters of tincture or fluid extract, 3 times a day for many weeks). I advise against taking sarsaparilla at all under these conditions.

The Formula That Works

To get the therapeutic benefits of sarsaparilla, look for organic sources of the herb, if available, and check for any amount of saponin content. Sarsaparilla is often sold as a whole herb, but my preference is, when possible, to get it freeze-dried in capsules or tablets. This form maintains a lot of the natural properties offered by nature. You can also find sarsaparilla in the following forms, again looking for whole herb, organically grown, listing saponin content.

Tincture:
    30–60 drops, 1–2 times per day (strength 1:1).

Capsules/Tablets:
    500 milligrams of root, 2–3 times a day.

Tea:
    2–6 grams of root brewed per day (sipped during the day).

Solid Extract:
150 milligrams, 1–2 times a day.

Is Sarsaparilla Right for Me?

Research on sarsaparilla certainly upholds its tonic reputation, but we see little to document the lore of its aphrodisiac properties. There is research to substantiate its use for gout, arthritis, psoriasis, ulcerative colitis and eczema (dermatitis). If you experience any of these conditions and feel the need of an all-around tonic to help you fight stress (which aggravates all of the listed conditions, by the way), sarsaparilla could certainly play a beneficial role in your overall therapeutic regimen.

L-ARGININE

In this section, we are going to talk about a different kind of substance—not an herb but an amino acid, a building block of protein found in various foods. Some of the foods that contain L-arginine have an aphrodisiac reputation, such as chocolate. In addition to chocolate, L-arginine can be found in seeds, peanuts, almonds and other nuts, in dairy foods, meat, fish, and poultry.

Ancient Roots

L-arginine doesn't have such ancient roots. In fact, it's hard to say just when L-arginine started getting a reputation as an aphrodisiac—possibly it began among weightlifters and bodybuilders, who took the amino acid for its ability to bulk up the muscles. Just a rumor that something works to enhance sex is enough to get lots of people trying it and talking about it. The buzz about L-arginine has been steady and positive.

How It Works

Chemically, L-arginine helps relax smooth-muscle contractions in the walls of the arteries and in the penis. This allows the arteries to dilate and circulation to increase. In the penis, this results in greater rigidity of erections. This amino acid is also crucial to sperm production and I have used it for treating infertility.

L-arginine is required for the constant replication of cells that takes place throughout the body, and its deficiency prevents the proper creation of cells. It is also needed for nitric oxide formation, which is documented to play a vital role in engorgement of the penile tissues and resulting sensation. One of the chemical actions that makes Viagra work is its ability to make nitric oxide available, enhancing the man's ability to attain an erection. Additionally, L-arginine plays crucial roles in the function and modulation of hormones such as insulin, growth hormones, and glucagon. L-arginine also stimulates the immune system and aids wound healing.

Research: Sexy Results

L-arginine has been studied for everything from tumor suppression to recovery from chemotherapy, and researchers have also documented its effects on sexual performance for men, leaving us to extrapolate the results for women. Here's the general rule: What's good for the penis, in terms of increased circulation and sensations, is good for the clitoris. Of the many studies conducted on this amino acid, there are some of particular interest to us:

- In a study at the University of Hawaii, reported in the Hawaii Medical Journal in 1998, 25 men who sought improved erectile functioning were giving a product called ArginMax for four weeks. Of the 21 men who completed the study, 88.9 percent reported improved erectile response, and 75 percent reported overall improvement in their sex life. No side effects were reported.

• A study conducted in France showed that L-arginine helped reduce erectile dysfunction stemming from both psychophysical and sexual asthenia (a medical term for weakness or debility).

• A Spanish study reported in *Clinical Science* in 1992 demonstrated that L-arginine helps maintain levels of nitric oxide, which is considered the main neurotransmitter in the corpus cavernosum, the long cylinders of tissue in the penis that fill up with blood to create an erection. L-arginine reverses the action of another amino acid that inhibits nitric oxide, resulting in enhanced penile blood flow.

• In 1991 the esteemed British medical journal *Lancet* reported a study that demonstrated L-arginine's positive effects on arterial blood flow in persons with elevated cholesterol. The amino acid reversed the constrictive effects of high cholesterol that decreased blood flow through the arteries. These results can be extrapolated to support the above-mentioned research on arginine's beneficial effect on erections.

Bottom line:

It looks to me like the research is taking L-arginine well into the realm of fact, at least where its effect on men is concerned. I give it four out of five stars, withholding the last star until we can see some research on its effects in women.

The Grandfather of Viagra

L-arginine works like the natural grandfather of Viagra, according to Steven Margolis, M.D. It is metabolized as nitric oxide, a gas that inflates the penis by allowing blood to flow in more easily. "It's about more than circulation," Dr. Margolis said. "Since the penis works on a hydraulic system, the gas itself has a dilation effect that is key to its success."

He learned about L-arginine's effects on arterial health at a seminar some years ago. "I kind of extrapolated a bit and tried it (for sexual dysfunction). I couldn't be sure it would work that way, but I never give a patient anything harmful, and there's a potential for good. Now you're starting to see it turn up in the literature, but I was a little ahead of them."

One of his patients, a pilot in his 40s, was taking Viagra but had to stop because of the side effect that gives vision a blue tint for several hours after taking a dose. That interfered with his ability to perform on the job. Dr. Margolis prescribed L-arginine instead. After two or three weeks of use, the patient reported "the exact same effect" as Viagra in attaining and maintaining an erection, without the negative side effects, and with the added bonus of reducing his high cholesterol. Not only that, a month's supply of L-arginine cost about the same as a single dose of Viagra.

Dr. Margolis' recommended dose is 1 gram, 3 times a day, which should begin to take effect in 2–3 weeks for a healthy person. He also uses L-arginine in combination with muira puama and avena sativa in a compound called Nutri-Man TNT.

Few Side Effects

Among healthy individuals, there are no known side effects with reasonable levels of L-arginine supplementation. As a side note, eating foods rich in lysine, such as most vegetables, legumes, fish, turkey, and chicken, can counter the effects of a therapeutic dosage of L-arginine. If these foods make up a large part of your diet, L-arginine may be less effective for you.

Not for Everyone

When taken at levels in the neighborhood of 30 grams per day (30,000 mg), L-arginine may decrease immune function, which is of particular concern in HIV, AIDS, and cancer patients. However, in the recommended moderate doses of 4000 mg a day, L-arginine can stimulate immune function.

When taken with ornithine (another amino acid used for muscle-building and to stimulate growth hormones), L-arginine can lead to increased growth hormone levels that, if elevated too greatly, may overload the pancreas, weakening it or creating a disease state. Those suffering from liver or kidney disease should exercise caution with L-arginine because it can put an extra burden on these two organs, which act as our body's filters of excess nutrients and toxins.

People with herpes simplex virus (HSV) should probably avoid the use of L-arginine. This virus requires the creation of protein structures rich in L-arginine in order to replicate. In addition, L-arginine stimulates the virus to reproduce itself more quickly.

The Formula That Works

According to a review of the research literature, an effective dose appears to be about 4000 mg per day. This can be taken as 2000 mg, two times a day, not with food.

Is L-arginine Right for Me?

During times of stress, particularly physical stress, our L-arginine levels can become deficient. By supplementing your diet with L-arginine during stressful times, you provide your system with a nutrient that is vital for physical and mental support, and this can help keep you feeling ready for action. If you are a body builder, or want to enhance your fertility, this is a particularly appropriate substance for you to try. Also, if you are experiencing any decreased circulation because of arterial blockage possibly caused by high cholesterol levels, L-arginine would be beneficial for you.

Among the roots, flowers, tree barks, and leaves we've talked about in this book so far, nothing is likely to cause you harm, although some, like yohimbe, require more caution than others. In our next chapter, we'll examine some alleged aphrodisiacs of great historical repute that should carry big warning labels.

9 BUYER BEWARE

After telling you all this time about the wonderful benefits of herbs, I now have to warn you that not everything natural is safe. There are herbs and other natural substances that can cause greater harm than good when used incorrectly or even when used at all. In this chapter, we will review three of those substances that have traditional, even legendary, uses as aphrodisiacs: Spanish fly, damiana, and ephedra. Experimenting with these is risky and can even be fatal. I have seen some patients who have tried so-called sexual enhancers on their own and suffered potentially serious effects. Fortunately, the worst symptoms they experienced were heart palpitations, dizziness, anxiety, and nausea. That they survived with no permanent injuries I can only attribute to youth, overall good health, and a whole lot of luck.

In "Buyer Beware," I will teach you to operate on a solid foundation of knowledge. Knowledge makes the difference between picking the wholesome mushroom and the poisonous one. Sometimes, the difference between a toxic plant and a medicinally beneficial one may be as simple as a slight variance in color. In other instances, the dosage is the factor. A good example of this is foxglove. This herb has offered humanity great benefits in the form of pharmaceuticals like digitalis, lanoxin, and digoxin, all of which help patients suffering from heart rhythm and contraction problems. But dosage is critical: just enough, and you live; too much or too little, and you die. Only a well-informed consumer can make the right choices.

Though this chapter is designed to offer you insight into the potential downsides of taking certain herbs, it nevertheless reinforces the fact that the majority of herbs can be consumed safely if: (1) the herb ingested is the right one for you and your unique health and biochemistry; and (2) the right dose is taken for a sufficient but not excessive period. In this chapter, we deal with substances that are unsafe for almost everyone, at almost any dose.

SPANISH FLY

This emerald green insect is actually a beetle rather than any sort of fly. Also called cantharides or cantharis, another folk name for it is the blister beetle. Its botanical name is bilingual: *Cantharis vesicatoria* or *Lytta vesicatoria*. In Latin, the word *vesica* means "blister," and *lytta* means "rage" in Greek. This storied insect lives in the southern parts of Europe. It grows to a length of ½ to ¾ inches long and ¼ of an inch wide, and emits a pungent odor. In its use as an aphrodisiac, it is crushed and eaten. Spanish fly's irritating effect on the urinary tract, which is manifested as a burning sensation in, and even erection of, the penis, must have been misconstrued as an aphrodisiac. But love is the last thing that will be on your mind if you try this age-old sexer-upper.

Ancient Roots

Spanish fly is probably the most famous aphrodisiac in Western history. Why it was dubbed "Spanish" is a mystery, since it was mentioned by the Greek physician Hippocrates and by the Roman historian Pliny. The Roman Empress Livia (58 B.C.–A.D. 29) allegedly dosed the food of family members with it and documented the resulting sexual improprieties for the purpose of blackmail. As we see, sex has also had a long history as political leverage.

While its use waned in the Middle Ages, it reappeared in the hands of none other than the Marquis de Sade, an infamous Frenchman of noble birth who made it his life's purpose to test the boundaries of sexual pleasure and pain— mostly his pleasure and others' pain. He reportedly offered candy spiked with Spanish fly to some prostitutes whom he had engaged for a flogging orgy. Instead of becoming sexually aroused, the women were made violently ill and the Marquis was charged and tried for poisoning them.

Spanish fly keeps reappearing in the popular culture as an aphrodisiac, mostly among urbanites, despite the fact that the FDA warned against its use in the early 1990s. One incident, however, has put a damper on its mystique. This scare occurred when a man consumed some Spanish fly that was tainted with strychnine. He ended up in the hospital with seizures, although he recovered. Popular attention has since turned to other natural products on the market, including some we discuss in this book. With such a persistent reputation dating back thousands of years, Spanish fly compels our examination.

How It Works

Spanish fly does indeed have a pronounced effect. It contains a substance called cantharidin that, when ingested in the form of crushed beetle, results in irritation of the entire urinary tract. The irritation results in increased blood flow to the area, and since the male urinary tract includes the penis, an erection occurs. It is easy to see how this particular symptom can be confused with sexual arousal, but enhanced desire is not the end result.

The erection response to Spanish fly isn't sexual any more than laughing when being tickled is funny. They are both reactions that are highly subject to misinterpretation. Additionally, an erection caused by Spanish fly is likely to be quite uncomfortable, since it is accompanied by a burning sensation. Remember, this so-called aphrodisiac is also referred to as the blister beetle.

We can only guess how this is supposed to work as a female aphrodisiac. A woman's urinary tract is not as closely entwined with her sexual organs, so she wouldn't experience any of the physiological effects that are associated with sexual excitement. She might confuse a burning sensation in her vagina with arousal, but certainly not for long.

Spanish fly does have some medicinal uses if applied very carefully. It can be used to remove warts and to treat urinary incontinence.

Research: Not So Sexy Results

I couldn't find any meaningful research on Spanish fly, and when you see the list of negative effects below, it is easy to see why no one thought it really necessary to conduct such research.

Side Effects/Interactions/Cautions

Spanish fly is extremely toxic either when taken orally or when it comes into contact with the skin. It has been reported to cause mental disturbance and may induce fits of rage. Other effects include heart palpitations, dizziness, and anxiety. One well-fed beetle could produce enough cantharidin to make you very sick; two beetles could be fatal. Poisoning can lead to inflammation of the kidneys and severe stomach and intestinal upset. In some cases, these symptoms can progress to circulatory collapse and death.

Not Right for Anybody

I can't think of any condition for which I would prescribe Spanish fly. There are many natural remedies other than the blister beetle that I would use for the few medical conditions it benefits. We can't diminish Spanish fly's legend, but we can leave it in the history books while we look to herbs and natural substances that nourish and heal the body while boosting our ability to be ready for love.

No Formula Works

There are Spanish fly products on the market, but the potential toxicity of this substance makes the lack of standardization especially dangerous. In my clinical opinion, there is no reason to take Spanish fly, and the risks are great, so the only formula for it that I can recommend is abstinence.

DAMIANA

This small shrub grows up to two feet. Its puts forth yellow flowers and its leaves are aromatic. It is found in dry, rocky climates, especially in the American southwest and in Mexico, but also in South America and the West Indies. The medicinal component is the leaf, harvested during the shrub's flowering season. Its botanical name is *Turnera diffusa*, also *Turnera aphrodiasica*. Unlike Spanish fly, damiana does enhance the sexual experience, but its side effects make this a potentially dangerous herb.

Ancient Roots

Damiana has been held in great esteem as an aphrodisiac since ancient times. Its popularity has remained strong over the course of the centuries, particularly in Mexico. It was used ritually by the Aztecs as a sexual stimulant. Medicinal uses have included treating depression, sterility, impotence, diabetes, and sexual imbalances. Folk uses have included treating asthma, bronchitis, neurosis, and various sexual disorders, according to James Duke, Ph.D., in his *Handbook on Medicinal Herbs* (1985). Damiana leaves have been used in the United States for the last hundred years or so, and it has gained popularity for its aphrodisiac effects in individuals who felt tired and lacked sufficient vitality. Its popularity spread across the Atlantic, where the Dutch herbalist E. F. Steinmetz reported in 1960 that damiana is renowned for its sex-enhancing qualities and positive effect on the sexual organs.

How It Works

Researchers haven't yet verified the folk uses of damiana, although the leaves are loaded with a variety of potentially beneficial chemicals. The leading contender so far is the presence of terpenes, or essential fragrant oils. The leaves also contain the substance arbutin, which has antimicrobial actions, alkaloids, and other potentially important compounds such as tannins and oils. Laboratory tests also suggest that damiana may also possess a slight progesterone-like effect, although this has yet to be substantiated in human studies. Though the research has not ferreted out the way it works, historically speaking it seems to have a following that warrants a closer look.

Research: Not So Sexy Results

While research has been conducted on the chemical makeup of damiana, there doesn't seem to be a body of research on its effects.

Side Effects/Interactions/Cautions

Among the side effects that may be experienced with damiana are diarrhea, vomiting, heart palpitations, anxiety, and possibly a manic-like state of euphoria. It should not be taken by those who are pregnant, breast feeding, or have heart, kidney, or blood pressure problems. Also, there is insufficient research to determine how damiana interacts with over-the-counter or prescription medications, but my educated guess is that damiana would have a very adverse effect on anyone taking anti-depressants or high blood pressure medication.

Not for Anyone Without
Medical Supervision

Damiana was used as a ritual drug by the Aztecs as much for its ability to alter the mental state as for any reputed aphrodisiac effect. This factor alone calls for great caution, and certainly medical supervision, in the use of this herb. While herbalists have also used damiana to increase urination (diuretic effect), to aid the digestion of fatty meals, and as a mild stimulant, my professional opinion is to work with your health care provider to find other natural substances that will help you achieve your goal of sexual enhancement. If you and your health care professional choose to try damiana, at the very least, make sure you are in good health, and are not taking any medication for depression, anxiety, psychological imbalances, blood pressure medicine, or heart medication.

The Formula That Works

According to folklore, damiana leaves must be harvested at a flowering stage of the plant's development to reap any reputed medicinal properties. However, this mandate is a flashing yellow light of "caution" in the use of this herb.

Such harvesting requires a level of expertise that is impossible to verify without standardization and testing of the resulting herbal product. Without that knowledge, it is impossible to say with any certainty what you are getting if you buy damiana at your local health food store.

You should not take this herb without working with a professional who has clinical experience with damiana, whether a doctor or an herbalist. The following list contains dosages that herbalists typically use for the crude herb, or raw leaf. Remember, more is *not* better, and if you experience any of the above effects, cease usage and contact your health care professional immediately.

Tea:
    1000 milligrams of leaves steeped in 8 ounces of hot water

Tincture:
    20–30 drops, 1–2 times a day

Capsules/Tablets:
    500 mg, 1–2 times a day

EPHEDRA

This shrub grows to a little over two feet in height and is native to China and surrounding Asian regions. Other species of ephedra grow in other countries, and each has varying degrees of active ingredients, but the Chinese version, *Ephedra sinica,* is the most widely used and researched. The medicinal parts are the young stems and roots, collected in the late summer or fall. While chemical elements of ephedra are processed into over-the-counter cold and allergy medications, those pharmaceutical products, and the raw herb itself, pose tremendous health risks if misused or abused.

Ancient Roots

Ephedra, also known in Chinese as Ma-Huang, is a powerful stimulant whose medicinal uses were identified in China nearly five thousand years ago. Traditional uses include treatment of hay fever, edema (swelling from water retention), arthritis, colds, asthma, bronchitis, and hives. It also had a reputation for rejuvenating the sexual function in the tired and elderly.

It was discovered by Western medicine in the early 1920s with research that showed ephedrine, an isolate of the plant, was indeed effective against the ailments for which the Chinese used it, especially respiratory problems like hay fever. The rest, as they say, is history, and today we can find hundreds of combinations of ephedrine and pseudoephedrine products for colds and allergies in drug stores and grocery stores worldwide. Such prescriptions account for millions of prescriptions each year.

How It Works

The active ingredient in ephedra is a chemical called ephedrine. It is a powerful stimulant, possessing as it does properties similar to one of our body's own stimulating chemicals, the hormone epinephrine (also known as adrenaline), that serves a critical role in each of our bodies as a neurotransmitter and a modulator of our metabolic rate and reactivity to stressful situations. The effects of ephedrine on the brain and central nervous system is similar to, but weaker than, that of amphetamine. Ephedrine has the ability to increase heart rate and work output and blood pressure. This stimulant action is the major reason for ephedra's reputation as an aphrodisiac and the major reason why this herb is so dangerous.

We know a lot about how ephedrine works because of the extensive research performed to get the U.S. pharmaceutical approval for it as an active ingredient in antihistamines used in cold and allergy medication. Even when the U.S. pharmaceutical version of ephedra is standardized and its dosage level well known, as is the case with the over-the-counter medications, ephedra derivates still pose extensive health risks to people with a variety of conditions or taking medications for diseases. Just take a look at the warning section of the packaging for these medications—this is not a harmless herb.

Though it is not clinically indicated for improvement of sexual function, many people experience the stimulant effect of ephedra as an aphrodisiac.

Medication Alert

One young man who was seeing me came in complaining of feeling edgy, and his heart was in his throat and pounding. When I took his pulse, it was racing over a hundred. "What's going on in your life," I asked him, looking for some sort of stressor that would account for his symptoms. "Are you up for a promotion? Got a new job? Seeing a new woman?" "I wish," he said. "Well are you eating anything new? Taking anything new?" Just some "natural decongestant" that he picked up at the health food store for a cold he was fighting. "Let me see," I said, suspiciously. Upon examining this "natural" remedy, I saw an ingredient listed as pseudoephedrine in a base of whole plant extract. He was taking enough of it to trigger such a strong stimulant effect that it was like he had adrenaline coursing through his body all the time. Without even moving his feet, this guy was experiencing the physical effects of a fight or flight response from some large animal with very sharp teeth. While this response can be a lifesaver, it isn't intended as a permanent state of being! Being in this state for days or weeks can cause an acute reaction, such as a heart attack. This is one natural substance that is not necessarily safe.

Though not the only concern regarding the use of ephedra products, lack of standardization of such a potentially powerful stimulant can lead to dramatic fluctuations of benefits and risks from product to product and batch to batch from even the same herbal supplier.

Research: Not So Sexy Results

While most research focuses on the respiratory benefits of ephedrine, there is some research on the aphrodisiac effect. For example, one double-blind study published in the Archives of General Psychiatry in 1998 found that ephedrine sulfate significantly increased sexual arousal in women. Results were measured two ways: by self-report of the 20 women tested, and by an instrument that measures, for example, vaginal muscle tone and responsiveness. It's interesting that although increased vaginal responses were measured, the women did not identify increased stimulus in their self-reports. These results pose a Zen-type question like the one about the tree falling in the forest: If women are aroused and they don't know it, does it matter?

Side Effects

Ephedra is an extremely powerful herb. Its ability to stimulate the heart, brain, respiratory system, and overall metabolism of the body can lead to heart attack, stroke, and death. Among the symptoms that are associated with toxic levels are dilated pupils, increased pulse, increased respiration, sweating, and others. If these symptoms occur while taking any ephedra product, you should seek immediate medical attention.

There is also the potential to become dependent on ephedra or its pharmaceutical extracts. The chance of becoming dependent increases with the duration of the use. Your risk for dependence will be different than the next person's, so pay no heed to the experience of your friend or your friend's friend.

Not for Everyone

There are certain conditions when neither the herb nor its pharmaceutical derivatives should ever be used:

- Aneurysm
- Anorexia
- Anxiety
- Diabetes
- Glaucoma
- Insomnia
- Heart Disease
- High Blood Pressure
- Hyperthryoid (High thyroid function)
- Nursing
- Pheochromocytoma (or other adrenal conditions)
- Pregnancy
- Prostate Enlargement
- Restlessness
- Stroke (or increased risk of)
- Ulcers

Ephedra should not be used with the following drugs and actually shouldn't be used with any drug without direct supervision of your physician:

- Alcohol—can lead to heart failure
- Caffeine—this combination may lead to over stimulation
- Guanethidine—can lead to increased metabolic stimulation
- Halothane—can alter heart rhythm

- Heart Glycosides—can disturb heart rhythm
- MAO Inhibitors—this combination can cause danger-
  ous over-stimulation
- Theophylline—increases nervous system stimulation
- Oxytocin—may lead to elevated blood pressure
- Secale Alkaloids—can result in increase blood pres-
  sure
- Viagra—the cumulative stimulation can be over-
  whelming and dangerous

The Formula That Works

Because this herb is so powerful, and the potential is great
for doing more harm than good, I do not recommend it and
feel it would be irresponsible to offer a recommended dose.
It should be noted that products readily available over-the-
counter containing pseudoephedrine deliver 30–60 mg per
dose. I don't believe ephedrine should be taken at such levels. In fact, ephedrine dosages are more commonly in the
range of 12.5 milligrams. Though it is tempting to try ephedra because of its stimulant effects, I would advise that other
natural products be used instead when striving to achieve
maximal sexual functioning.

Is Ephedra Right for Me?

Ephedra is the original natural source for pharmaceutical
compounds that are available both over-the-counter and by
prescription. It has been used for numerous conditions
including: asthma, nasal congestion, respiratory congestion,
and temporary weight loss. Since the risk is high relative to
the lack of strong and safe use as a self-prescribed aphrodisiac, I would use ephedra only for the well-researched respiratory uses. If there happen to be any simultaneous aphrodisiac effects, just enjoy them (if you feel well enough!) until

your medical condition is gone and you stop taking the medication.

Be a Conscientious Consumer

The herbal consumer is frequently bombarded with all the wonders of the potential benefits of the various herbal products and blends. Usually, the products are both safe and, to varying degrees, effective. Of course, the real challenge occurs when having to decide if buying a product is worth the time, money, and on some occasions, the experiment.

When reviewing Spanish fly, damiana, and ephedra, we touched upon some of the most popular herbs that the potential consumer should view with great caution, and definitely discuss with their physician, before considering any experimentation. As a clinician and as author of a book on the interaction of drugs and natural products, I approach the mixing of drugs and herbs with a degree of caution. So, when thinking about taking any herb or supplement in your pursuit of optimal health or sexual experience, knowledge is key to finding the balance of the right herb for you at the right dosage. In the case of these three, I would have to say, "none of the above." There are ample choices throughout this book of herbs that nourish you and spark your sexual desire.

10 EVERYDAY CHOICES FOR BETTER SEX

A book called *Better Sex Naturally* just wouldn't be complete without exploring the myths and facts that surround the dietary and lifestyle choices that can spice up your sex life. In the preceding chapters, we have reviewed some of the most popular and effective herbal treatments used to stimulate sexual functioning directly, as well as those that act indirectly to support the critical parts of our body needed to enjoy that stimulation. Now, we'll take a quick look at some basic lifestyle information to help you live life to the fullest, in and out of the bedroom.

As we discussed in the first chapter of this book, having sex at all, let alone great sex, requires many systems in our body to work in concert. Our heart has to pump blood faster and harder throughout the body, including the sex organs, because, to varying degrees, sex is an aerobic workout. Our nervous system must send the appropriate messages to have each of our erogenous areas and organs working in sync, and, of course, the brain needs sufficient stimuli to help with artistic interpretation and allow full appreciation of the performance. Beyond the heart and nervous system, our hormonal balance influences our ability to follow the script. We need all this and more for the show to go on. The right balance of food, rest, and activity serve as the supporting cast for vibrant health and enjoyment of all aspects of life, including sex.

As we address the basics of a healthy and well-rounded diet and lifestyle, think of these recommendations as mile markers on your journey to optimal health and sex. Of course, the sooner you begin, the quicker you may reap the fruits of your labor. Making the right choices enough of the time is indeed a labor; take it from a physician who works with all his patients on diet and lifestyle changes. The key to optimal health is making these changes slowly, integrating them into your daily life. It also helps to find a partner to make these changes with. In my mind, there is no better person with whom to embark on this endeavor than with your life partner. The key, of course, is moderation. The 100% perfect diet and lifestyle might help you live to the ripe old age of 120, but it is important to have fun along the way.

You've heard these tips before, and though they may not have been tied specifically to sex, I think you've learned now that everything that affects your health also affects your sex life. Learning to make new choices is like buying an insurance policy for a lifetime of good sex. Just think of it as you would your car; you enjoy driving your car, and as a result you carry insurance on it just in case it gets damaged. Well, there is no ready replacement for your health, so following these guidelines is a way to protect the most valuable commodity you own: yourself.

Move It!

Probably the most fun exercise you get is sex, and you can make that even better by getting a little every day—exercise, that is. The experts tell us only one out of every five Americans exercises regularly. Those who don't usually cite lack of time or energy as excuses, but this is really a matter of priorities. What's really important to you? Sex, of course, because you're reading this book, but what else?

Whether the answer is worldly possessions, like cars and homes, or spiritual things like family and friends, they are all best enjoyed when you are in good health, and exercise is crucial to your health. Remember when you were a kid and you could hardly stop running around because you had so much energy? When I was a kid, I would play outside until my parents called me in each evening, then drag my feet all the way inside. Well now, what happened to all that energy? Getting older is part of it, but it's a case of use it or lose it— the more you move, the more energy you will have. You can trigger that cycle again, now, no matter your age or state or health. All of us know people of our age or older who can run us into the ground. Any lack of energy you may be experiencing is probably due to not staying fit, not getting enough sleep, or just dealing with too much stress.

Physical activity is the answer to all three of these! There is no single better way to rid your body of stress than finding an activity that you enjoy and doing it. Frustration will melt away and so will a few extra inches. One of my patients with high blood pressure began complaining of being tired. I told him to take a leisurely walk for 20–30 minutes each morning before he went off to work. He followed the prescription for 30 days before he came back to see me, and not only did he begin to feel and look substantially better, his blood pressure returned to normal and his stress levels all but disappeared. He also reported sleeping like a log.

Starting a low-impact, low-stress exercise routine such as walking or swimming can help you get your energy level back on track. It will also improve the quality of your sex life. You may be able to convince yourself that feeling tired, stressed, and being out of shape doesn't affect your sexual performance and enjoyment, but I'll bet your partner has a different opinion!

Sleep Well and Prosper

Millions of Americans are walking around every day in a semi-stupor from lack of sleep. Researchers have linked sleep deprivation to serious health concerns such as depression, chronic fatigue, and other degenerative conditions, at least in part. Any of these conditions, let alone lack of sleep, will certainly have a detrimental effect on your sex life as well. Sleep is when the body and mind recuperate, heal, and grow. Researchers have actually linked chronic sleep deprivation with shorter and less healthy lives. A common complaint from partners of the sleep-deprived is: "We made love and s/he was out like a light." Beyond this type of annoyance, there lurks a larger problem. If you have ever stayed up all night long cramming for an exam, or just having fun, you will remember that reality began to become distorted, blurred around the edges, or, at the very least, a little fuzzy. This is no way to go through life!

There are many reasons why people don't get enough sleep, but no matter which reason is yours, it's a matter of priorities again. I believe sleep is important enough to schedule in your day planner—eight hours of it. You say you don't have time for eight hours of sleep, yet the paradox is, if you made this a priority you might find your waking time more productive, leaving you more time to sleep!

Equally as important as quantity of sleep is quality of sleep. The REM (rapid eye movement) stage of sleep is when dreams occur. Dreams serve as a way to process and integrate whatever happens in our daily lives. It has been said that it is our dreams that keep us sane. Some people swear they do not dream, but if you reach the REM stage, you will dream. If you don't remember your dreams consistently, that may be an indicator of depression; also, researchers say those who do not remember their dreams may find their creativity is diminished. Some nutritionally oriented physicians suggest that not remembering one's dreams is often a sign of vitamin B complex deficiency.

If you feel you aren't getting enough sleep, try making this a priority and see what a difference it makes in your life. Like many pieces of advice, this is easier said than done, but here are a few tips my patients have shared with me over the years:

Insomniacs.
Get into a regular exercise routine and don't read or watch television in bed (the mind should associate the bed only with sleep—and sex!)

Busy bees.
Get into a routine of going to bed at the same time, plus or minus 30 minutes. Literally put it in your day planner, or better yet, do not schedule past a certain time for either work or social activities. Realize that you might not get everything done today, but tomorrow will come, and you want to be awake for it.

Worriers.
Bring a pad and pencil to bed and put it on the night stand. Write down all your unfinished business, and if something else pops into your mind later, write down one or two key words to put your mind at ease. One of my patients tells me that when work starts spiraling around in her head as she tries to sleep, she reminds herself that the very best thing she can do at that moment is sleep to be ready for it tomorrow.

Night stalkers.

If you are getting up in the night several times to urinate, don't drink any liquids 2–3 hours prior to bed. If you are a man, discuss this issue with your doctor and try saw palmetto. If you get leg cramps that wake you up and you are healthy and not on other medications, think about supplementing your diet with calcium or magnesium. And for those with restless, twitchy legs, folic acid can work wonders.

◆ ◆ ◆

If you are among the millions of the awake and sleepy during the day, caffeine is not the solution; it perpetuates the cycle of sleep difficulty by preventing a good night's sleep. Try to get more sleep, and if that doesn't work, talk to your doctor about testing for anemia, checking your thyroid function, and getting some simple blood work done. I do this for myself and my patients once a year. Annually, I suggest that they have a couple of tests called a chemistry panel (measuring blood sugar, liver and gallbladder enzymes, cholesterol, minerals like calcium and magnesium, and thyroid function), and a complete blood count (or CBC) that will check your immune system and see if you are anemic. It would be a shame if you tried one of the *Better Sex Naturally* tips and weren't fully awake to enjoy the results!

Food Is Medicine

A basic premise of naturopathic medicine is borrowed from the ancient Greek physician Hippocrates, who said, "Let your food be your medicine, and let your medicine be your food." I subscribe wholeheartedly to that philosophy and tell you that food is, indeed, our best medicine. Ever since we were kids, we have been told that food provides the building blocks for a strong and healthy body. As we now know, our parents were right about this. Not only is a good diet crucial to a growing body, it is equally important in preventing the development of conditions that can negatively affect our health, and even our sex lives. With healthy eating, the majority of health problems that take a toll on your sex life—and your life in general—can be avoided totally, or at least postponed dramatically.

A good diet, in my mind, emphasizes moderation and variety. Dessert and occasional indulgences are fine in the context of mostly healthy choices. After all, the spirit of a nutritious eating plan is to improve the quality of one's life. If your diet makes you miserable, it would be hard to argue that your quality of life has improved!

Personally, I recommend that my patients who want a long and active life, including great sex in their golden years, observe the following guidelines: Eat small meals, and make sure not to overeat. Chew your food well and try not to hurry through your meals, because it lessens your ability to digest and absorb nutrients. Don't drink very much liquid with your meal because it dilutes your digestive juices, decreasing your body's ability to maximize food value. Also, by chewing your food well and not drinking liquids with your meals, there is less bloating, gas, and gastrointestinal complaints.

I suggest that carbohydrates make up 50–60% of the calories in our diet, with most of those being complex carbohydrates. Protein should make up 20–30% of the calories we ingest, and should be derived primarily from beans, legumes, soy, and nuts other than peanuts, with some fish and lean meat. Fats should be minimally saturated or hydrogenated, and ideally come from vegetables, grains, and nuts. Meat is a source of saturated fat, so it should be eaten sparingly. It is also important to remember that frying and heating your cooking oils can change their chemical structure, converting them to hydrogenated oils, which increases their potential to cause damage in the body.

Food for Life

There are hundreds of books written about which foods you should eat and which you should avoid. Some of my patients get fed up with trying to keep them straight or to make sense of the high-protein diet versus the high-carbohydrate diet. Instead of trying to list all the foods that are good or bad for your body, let's talk about some easy-to-remember guidelines.

Fiber

In spite of the volumes of popular articles on this key dietary ingredient, I still get questions from my patients about what fiber is, exactly. Fiber typically refers to the part of plants that is not readily digestible, offers little direct nutritional value, and adds bulk to the diet. It is found primarily in unprocessed, plant-based foods. Let's put it this way: A home gardener could not go wrong walking out to the vegetable patch and grabbing something to eat. You know you're eating fiber if you have to chew a lot. Take bread, for example: The whole grain variety is chewy, which, by the way, requires muscle exercise that burns calories; white bread melts in your mouth. For the creative reader, saltwater taffy and caramel, though they require chewing, don't count as fiber!

So, what does fiber have to do with good sex? Fiber improves digestion, keeps the intestines healthy, and, when not overdone, lessens gas attacks which can make you easier to be around for your partner. Some people complain of gas when they add more fiber to their diet, but that is usually because their system has become unused to processing it in healthy amounts. Also, fiber lessens the risk of colon cancer, helps lower cholesterol levels, and helps balance out hormones. Often, hormones such as estrogen and progesterone that are excreted into the intestines are reabsorbed by the body, leading to their excessive build up in the blood and resulting in everything from mood swings to physical imbalances, such as fluid retention, breast cancer, and tenderness, including premenstrual tenderness.

Fresh Fruits and Veggies

Fresh fruits and vegetables are an abundant source of antioxidants, substances that offer protection against heart disease and cancer, and many other valuable nutrients. The benefits provided by eating the recommended 5–7 servings of fruits and vegetables per day are indeed amazing. They include a lowered chance of ailments such as high blood pressure, heart disease, and certain types of cancer. Other benefits are improved bowel function, an improved complexion, a healthier heart overall, and generally increased energy and stamina. One more benefit of adding fruits and vegetables to your diet is that by focusing on these ultra-healthy foods, you have less room for the unhealthy ones, such as fatty or fried foods. Many of us have seen the commercials touting the benefits of juicing. Whether you eat them or drink them, one of your goals should be to get those 5–7 servings a day. If your idea of a vegetable is ketchup, start with a few small servings and work up to the recommended amount.

Meat: Lean and Organic

There is nothing wrong with being an omnivore, just as long as you do it right. Meat should be a "bit-player" in your cast of foodstuffs, rather than the star. One should focus on chicken and turkey, not fried, and ideally without the skin. If possible, choose organic meats to spare yourself the buildup of hormones, antibiotics, and other additives found in the meat at your grocery store. Incorporate deep cold-water fish, like cod and halibut, into your diet. This type of fish is a rich source of a "good" type of fat, called omega–3 fatty acids, which bolster the immune system, lessen inflammation, and can actually help ward off heart disease.

These dietary recommendations are goals for you to work toward, incorporating them gradually into your life. Don't try to overhaul your diet all at once. Those types of changes seldom stick, and it's better to make slow and steady changes, allowing them to become a normal part of your eating pattern. But it is important to start making those changes now!

Contraindicated

With all you are doing to improve your sexual experience and your overall health, there are several routine behaviors that will sabotage your efforts.

Smoking

Great sex takes a lot of lung capacity, and nothing has a bigger impact on your lung capacity than smoking. Not only that, nicotine constricts the blood vessels and can lessen blood flow to sex organs, diminishing the responsiveness of erectile tissue, the penis and the clitoris, and vaginal lubrication. And even if you can live with those effects, see if this one gets your attention: The U.S. Surgeon General reports that smoking is the *single most important controllable risk factor* for heart disease and cancer, the #1 and #2 killers of Americans. These will put a big crimp in your sex life, but the good news is that this risk factor is controllable. It's not easy, but it's controllable. Kicking nicotine is one of the hardest things to do; that's what research shows and that's what my patients tell me. One shared this joke with me about it, "Doc, why is it that smokers have low back pain?" I tried a few medically based guesses, but you probably know the real answer. "Because everyone is always on your back to quit smoking."

As hard as quitting is, you can take comfort in knowing

that 40 million Americans have done it, probably not the first time they tried, and certainly not without some pain, but they have proven it can be done. There are some natural substances that can help. I often recommend niacinamide (a form of vitamin B), drinking oat tea (*Avena sativa*), homeopathic stop-smoking formulas, and stress reduction techniques. One former smoker shared a tip with me that may work for you: When you want more than anything in the world to take a deep drag on a cigarette, try that same deep breathing without the nicotine. Deep breathing reduces stress all by itself, and lowering your stress level can diminish the need to smoke. She said drinking a lot of water helped, too, just from the behavioral standpoint of jumping up and doing something when she wanted to light up. Water is a good choice, rather than coffee or caffeinated soda, which can aggravate your stress levels. Also be sure to avoid any situations that you know trigger your desire to smoke, such as being with friends when they are smoking. A favorite technique my patients have enjoyed using is imagining how they are going to spend the money they save from not smoking, and then going out and buying something nice for themselves.

Rich Meals

So you're going out for a romantic dinner to set the stage for a night of love. If you want the night to fulfill its promise, make sure you steer clear of fatty and rich culinary delights. Digesting those meals is a lot of work for your system, and blood gets rerouted from sexual regions to the digestive tract. It also appears that eating a fatty meal actually causes blood vessels to constrict, lessening the ability of the body as a whole to get sufficient oxygen and energy to sustain exertion. And these are just the short-term problems! A lifetime of such food can mean a short life.

Alcohol

A little wine, perhaps? Well, just a little. Though alcohol has been an age-old stand-by to lessen sexual inhibition, the exact dosage at which you loosen up but can still function optimally is not listed anywhere on the bottle. It's very easy to cross the line between that warm, glowing feeling and that "wasn't there something we were going to do?" feeling. Also, as was mentioned in the "Especially for Men" chapter, alcohol can affect long term performance and can have an addictive effect over time.

Most of us violated some or all of these guidelines many times in our lives. Youth serves us well as a buffer, but I promise you that time and our indiscretions will catch up with us sooner or later. Use the advice from this chapter to stave off that day of reckoning, and keep your sex life simmering. And, for extra sizzle, try the reputed aphrodisiac foods listed below.

Fun Foods to Fuel Lovers

Herbs are just part of the menu for better sex naturally, and they cross the line into everyday foods more often than you might think. Take garlic and onion for example—food or herb? Both! The ancient Greeks and Egyptians thought of them as aphrodisiacs. Though research has yet to prove the effectiveness of onion to rev one's engine, so has it failed to look at many empirically proven herbal remedies. I would be the last one to argue with the ancient Arabs, who created the numbers that we use today, the Egyptians, who built pyramids we would struggle to duplicate, the Greeks, who created awe-inspiring monuments and discovered mathematical principles that govern our modern life, and the other founding cultures of our current civilization. When it comes to sex, we must assume that ancient cultures can teach us some truly practical things. Since we are all here only because our ancestors figured out how to keep their sex drive going during famines, plagues, and the intermittent saber tooth tiger chase, we must tip our hats to them. You can do some research yourself with this menu to see whether these foods fuel your sexual appetite.

Asparagus

There's an ancient medical concept, called the Doctrine of Signatures, which suggests the way a plant looks reflects its potential use. With that in mind, it doesn't take a lot of imagination to contemplate the possible use of asparagus as a sexual aid. In fact, ancient Arabs and Greeks cultivated it for use as an aphrodisiac. This usage is supported by some herbalists who believe that it works as a result of its ability to stimulate the urinary tract and related tissues.

Betel Nut

It has been suggested by some early texts found in India that consuming these berries, also referred to as nuts, will bring feelings of love to the surface.

Celery

Though we lack any scientific validation of its benefits, celery is believed to increase the potential for arousal. We don't quite understand how this works yet, but the empirical data is slowly gathering momentum behind this simple and common food.

Chocolate

It is said that the great Italian lover Casanova was a big fan of chocolates. In the 1800s, doctors actually prescribed chocolate to help their patients in the romance department. Thus, romance, chocolate, and Valentine's Day are virtually inseparable.

Fennel

The ancient Egyptians and Greeks looked to fennel to achieve peak sexual arousal. The leaves and seeds of this flavorful plant were used in festivals and celebrations.

Grapes

Fermented or unfermented, grapes were held in high esteem by the ancient Greeks. Both were thought to be sexually stimulating. Dionysus, the Greek god of wine, was also the god of fertility. We know now that wine and grape juice support a healthy heart and offer bioflavonoids and antioxidants that protect our bodies against conditions such as heart disease and cancer.

Onions

Onions appear to be one of the chosen foods of the ancients. For centuries the Greeks, Romans, Egyptians, and Arabs have looked to onions to spice up more than their food. It is said that, during the time of the Pharaohs, Egyptian priests were forbidden to eat onions lest this food lead them astray from their vows of celibacy. The ancient Greeks, Romans, and Arabs all used onion in certain recipes as an aphrodisiac. The infamous Hindu books on the art of making love make numerous mentions of this earthbound plant. And let's not forget the French, who have something of a reputation in this field. One French tradition is to serve onion soup to newlyweds the morning after the wedding, reputedly to restore and revitalize them after their first night of passion.

If you've got a strong stomach, here's a recipe from the ancients that you could try: Press out fresh onion juice and mix one part of the juice with two parts honey. Then warm the solution until it has concentrated a little, let it cool, and use when needed.

Oysters

It is thought that oysters first got their reputation as an aphrodisiac from the myth of the Greek goddess of love, Aphrodite, riding an oyster shell to the surface of the sea. You can see how the two elements, love and oysters, would become associated. Oysters next hit it big at the height of the Roman Empire. Some reports suggest that oysters were worth their weight in gold to the Roman elite, who prized them for their ability to heighten sexual pleasure. A more modern story is that of famous ladies' man Casanova's supposed love of raw oysters.

Whether modern science will prove the sexy effects of oysters, only time will tell. Yet the potential seems to be present, if nutrient content counts for anything. Oysters are known to be high in numerous minerals, foremost being zinc and iodine. Zinc is essential for the production of testosterone, the major sex drive hormone in both men and women. Zinc also supports sperm formation.

Pine Nuts

Another purported aphrodisiac is pine nuts. Historically, the cultures surrounding the Mediterranean were getting big results from these little nuts some 2000 years ago. One reported recipe used a mix of honey, almonds, and pine nuts. This blend was used for three days prior to seeing its full effect. One might explain the effectiveness of such a concoction by analyzing its rich nutrient value. If I were to make a clinical guess as to why such a formula would be effective, my assessment would rely on the high L-arginine and zinc content, and the carbohydrate/protein balance. The arginine would help both male and female erectile tissue to react more quickly and be more responsive, increasing sensitivity and function. The zinc would support testosterone production. And, finally, the blend of the quick energy of the car-

bohydrates derived from the honey with the staying power
of the time released energy of protein could help both the
sprinter and marathoner.

Quince

This fruit has been used widely throughout the region of
the Mediterreanean. The ancient Greeks and Romans both
dedicated it to their goddesses of love, Aphrodite and
Venus, respectively. Quinces also have been used traditionally in wedding ceremonies and are believed to instill happiness and contentment amongst married couples. The color
and the sweet fragrance that springs from the quince has led
some historians and biblical scholars to believe that, since it
appears to be indigenous to the region believed to contain
the Garden of Eden, the quince may have been the forbidden fruit that tempted Eve.

Truffles

The Romans believed that truffles had strong aphrodisiac
properties. Though modern use of truffles as a potent aphrodisiac has waned, they are still regarded as sensuous in a culinary sense. If you have an opportunity, why not try them and
see for yourself?

Walnuts

Ancient Romans reportedly used walnuts in fertility ritu-
als. Some believed in the aphrodisiac properties of these
nuts, and they tossed them at weddings the way we toss rice.
I hope the newlyweds had protective headgear!

Bon Appetit!

It is fitting that we wrap up this book of herbs for better
sex with the above menu of aphrodisiac foods, because life is
a banquet, and sex is one of its most savory dishes. Both food

and herb, wherever you draw the line between them, are the fuel not only for your sex life, but for your whole life, and if your search for better sex leads to better health and well-being, then that's the sauce on top! Now you are equipped with the knowledge to begin to nourish your entire being for all the excitement you can stand in every area of your life. Sex is a great barometer of quality of life, and as your strength and stamina increase, I wish for you the joy of a healthy life and better sex, naturally!

Appendix A: PUTTING IT ALL TOGETHER—AN HERBAL SHOPPING LIST

As we have discovered, there are many herbs that can be used to boost your sexual desire and performance. So, the question is: Where does one begin? Here are some tips to help you put together an herbal shopping list that is right for you. First I will provide some useful tips on being a conscientious herbal consumer. Then in Section I I'll discuss general recommendations for both men and women to increase sexual stamina, endurance, and blood flow to sex organs and more. Sections II and III follow, with an overview of Single Herb Favorites for Men and Single Herb Favorites for Women. Finally, I will give you some useful guidelines for purchasing herbal combinations and provide suggestions that I have used with great success to energize, revitalize, and peak overall performance in my patients.

When Buying Herbs

With the scores of herbal products available in natural food stores, supermarkets, and pharmacies today, you know that making a sound choice can be a daunting experience. Here are some simple pointers to selecting wholesome products that will nourish your body and help you achieve your goals.

Unprocessed Herbs vs. Extracts

Keep in mind that there are two distinct approaches to choosing herbs, whether to enhance your sex life or to improve your overall health. One is to purchase an herb in its raw or unprocessed form. This approach represents the classic use of herbal medicine by indigenous cultures who incorporated herbs into their diets, hence the concept of "herbal medicine as food." Some herbs are powerful enough on their own to be used in this fashion. Among the herbs we cover in this book that fall into this category are ginseng, ashwaganda, muira puama, black cohosh, and dong quai. The second approach developed from our ability to tinker with nature by concentrating the active ingredients in herbs to make powerful extracts. In an extract, an herb's potency is distilled into a form many times more concentrated than the raw herb. An example of this is standardized gingko extract, which, as we mentioned in the gingko chapter, is concentrated into a form equivalent to 50 times as potent as the leaf from which it is made. Other examples from this book are saw palmetto and pygeum. You can tell an extract when you see the ratio for the concentrate on a label. A 1:2 concentration is twice as strong as the raw herb; 1:6 is six times as concentrated; 1:50 is 50 times as concentrated. In my opinion, one form is no better than the other. The best choice is the one that works to address the underlying cause of a problem without harming the patient.

Looking at Labels

When you compare products, look on the label for "certified organic" or "wildcrafted." This means the manufacturers did not use chemical pesticides and/or herbicides on their products. This is an important standard to hold to any medicinal product you consume. The last thing you want and need when optimizing your health and sex life is additional chemicals in your body. In fact, certain chemicals used in agricultural processes have been linked to causing hormonal imbalances in men and women.

Also make sure that the manufacturer adheres to "true labeling," which means that it lists all the ingredients and dosages in an accurate fashion. The sales person at your local health food store or the customer service representative at the manufacturer can help clarify a company's standards. You can also look for the NNFA label on products. This means that a company belongs to the National Nutritional Foods Association, an organization that is comprised of product manufacturers who are actively pursuing self-regulation and creating comprehensive guidelines for quality.

SINGLE HERB SHOPPING LIST

Section I: Recommendations for Both Men and Women
Herbs/Nutrients that Can Increase Blood Supply to Sex Organs and More

I commonly prescribe one or more of the following herbs or amino acids for my male and female patients who want to improve blood flow to sex organs, improve overall circulation, and improve overall sense of wellness and stamina.

Arginine
Capsules/Tablets:
1000–2000 milligrams, 2 times a day away with a light meal or snack

Gingko
Capsules/Tablets:
   40–60 milligrams, 3 times a day (24% standardized which is 50:1)
Tinctures:
   30–60 drops, 3 times a day (standardized to 24% if possible)
Tea:
   (Offers less immediate effects: I recommend the above forms)

Yohimbe*
Capsules/Tablets:
   15–25 milligrams per day (taken in divided doses)
Tinctures:
   Dosage varies greatly; follow the directions given on the package
Tea:
   (Typically not available in this form commercially)

*When using yohimbe, it is important to remember that it can interact with certain medications and should not be used by people who have high blood pressure, diabetes, and other conditions listed in Chapter 5. Yohimbe should be taken only under the guidance of a physician. Since the products in natural food stores vary greatly in terms of strength, I suggest you obtain this herb by prescription from your doctor.

Herbs Useful for Increasing Endurance and Sexual Energy
   I have used these herbs to help men and women spice up their sex lives and enhance the duration and depth of their sexual performance.

Aswaghanda
Capsules/Tablets:
   1000 milligrams, 1–2 times a day
Tinctures:
   60–90 drops, 2–3 times a day
Tea:
   1000–1500 milligrams, 2–3 times a day

Ginseng
Capsules/Tablets:
   (standardized) 10 milligrams of ginenoside Rg1 (1:2 ratio of Rg1:Rb1)
   (unprocessed) 500–1000 milligrams, 2–3 times a day
Tinctures:
   500–1000 milligrams, 1–2 times a day
Tea:
   1 tablespoon cooked in 6 ounces of water 2–3 times a day

Muira Puama
Capsules/Tablets:
   250 milligrams, 3 times a day (ideally 6:1 concentrate)
Tinctures:
   Not readily available
Tea:
   Not readily available

Wild Oats
Capsules/Tablets:
   1000 milligrams, 2–4 times a day
Tinctures:
   30–60 drops, 2–4 times a day
Tea:
   1 tablespoon per 8 ounce cup 2–4 times a day

Section II: Herb Favorites for Men
Herbs that Help Maintain Overall Male Reproductive Health and Sexual Energy

The following herbs all have both rich traditional use history and proven clinical effectiveness that demonstrate their ability to increase sexual performance directly and indirectly by keeping the equipment tuned-up. These herbs can provide support to the prostate and reproductive tract while increasing your chances of eking out a little more horsepower from each piston. Over the course of two weeks to two months you should notice improved performance and a general sense of wellbeing. You should also experience better overall male reproductive health, increased urine flow, and diminished need to make bathroom trips during the middle of the night.

Damiana
(Note that I have also included this herb in Chapter 9: Buyer Beware. Use it only under medical supervision.)
Capsules/Tablets:
   500 milligrams, 1–2 times a day
Tinctures:
   20–30 drops, 1–2 times a day
Teas:
   1000 milligrams in 8 ounces of water

Flower Pollen
Capsules/Tablets:
   60–120 milligrams, 2–3 times a day

Pygeum
Capsules/Tablets:
   100–250 milligrams, 1–2 times a day
   (Standardized 14% terpenes/beta sitosterol/0.5% n-docosanol)

Tincture:
   (Not readily available or used)
Tea:
   (Not readily available)

Sarsaparilla
Capsules/Tablets:
   500 milligrams, 2–3 times a day
Tinctures:
   60–120 drops, 2 times a day
Tea:
   2–6 grams in 8–16 ounces of water sipped on throughout day

Saw Palmetto
Capsules/Tablets:
   160 milligrams, 2–3 times a day (85–95% fatty acids/liposterols)
Tincture:
   5–6 milliliters per day (taken in 2 separate doses)
Tea:
   2–3 grams per 8 ounces of water, 2 times a day

Urtica
Capsules/Tablets:
   300–500 milligrams, 3–4 times a day
Tincture:
   30 drops, 3–4 times a day
Tea:
   1 Tablespoon, 3–4 times a day

Herbs and Nutrients to Enhance Erectile Rigidness
There is not a guy around who, somewhere along the way, hasn't expected more from his performance, or who has

wondered what he could do to make sure things keep working as well as they have been. Arginine and the first two
herbs discussed below are particularly worth giving a try. On
the other hand, I would keep yohimbe in the wings, since
there are increased risks for side effects, and this herb really
should be prescribed by your doctor. If by chance you happen to suffer from cold hands or feet, poor circulation, or a
little slippage in the memory department, arginine, gingko,
and muira puama might just provide an added benefit as
well.

Arginine
Capsules/Tablets:
   1000–2000 milligrams, 2 times a day away from meals

Gingko
Capsules/Tablets:
   40–60 milligrams, 3 times a day (24% standardized,
which is 50:1)
Tinctures:
   30–60 drops, 3 times a day (standardized to 24% if possible)
Tea:
   (Offers less immediate effects: I recommend the above
forms)

Muira Puama
Capsules/Tablets:
   250 milligrams, 3 times a day (ideally 6:1 concentrate)
Tinctures:
   Not readily available
Tea:
   Not readily available

Yohimbe
Capsules/Tablets:
    15–25 milligrams per day (taken in divided doses)
Tinctures:
    4–8 drops, 3 times a day
Tea:
    (Typically not available in this form commercially)

Section III: Herb Favorites for Women:
Herbs that Support Female Sexual Balance and Vitality

These herbs have been used for centuries by indigenous cultures and all continue to enjoy great popularity today. Each of these herbs has the ability to tone the body and help it self-regulate its hormonal balance. Both of these activities are crucial to a woman's sexual health and vitality. My patients who have experienced PMS and menopausal symptoms, and who are also wishing to improve their sexual enjoyment and health, often report good results when using these herbs. Even if you haven't had any symptoms of PMS or menopause, these herbs can still be helpful, but you may also want to try the general recommendations in Section I of this appendix.

Black Cohosh
Capsules/Tablets:
    (unprocessed) 500 mg, 1–2 times a day
    (standardized) 250 mg, 2–4 times per day (2.5% triterpene glycosides)
Tincture:
    1 teaspoon, 2–3 times a day
Tea:
    500 mg, 2–4 times a day

Dong Quai

Capsules/Tablets:
   1000 mg, 3–4 times a day
Tincture:
   45–60 drops, 2–3 times a day
Tea:
   1 Tablespoon per cup of hot water, 3–4 times a day

Wild Yam

Capsules/Tablets:
   500–1000 mg, 3 times a day
Tincture:
   30–60 drops, 2–3 times a day
Tea:
   ½ Tablespoon, 1–2 times a day

Herbal Formulas

As you know, besides the dozens of single herbs on the store shelves, there are also scores of herbal formulas available today. Naturopathic physicians use herbal combinations quite often and quite successfully. When choosing a formula we make sure that each medicinal component individually contributes to the effectiveness and safety of the product and also works in synergy with the other ingredients. Herbal combinations not only bring relief for the conditions or symptoms for which they are specifically designed, but like single herbs, they also promote a general feeling of sound health.

Labels, Again

When looking at the barrage of combinations, keep the following in mind: When you see a laundry list of ingredients, it means that there is less of each ingredient per capsule than a formula that has only a few select ingredients. So, as you select a product, you have the option of picking a precise formula with higher concentrations of each ingredient or opting for a broader approach that counts primarily on the synergy of the ingredients for its effect. If you know what you hope to accomplish specifically with a formula (like increasing blood flow to enhance sexual function), picking a product with only four-to-six ingredients that specifically support that goal (like gingko, arginine, and muira puama) would probably be better than a list of eighteen ingredients in smaller quantities that represent more of a shotgun approach. Remember, too, that *Better Sex Naturally* certainly can help you make sound choices since you now have an insider's insight into the benefits of each herb and how it might harmonize with your body.

Added Nutrients

As you look at various herbal formulas, you often will find minerals and vitamins included in the blends. You can tell a lot about a formula's quality by the types and forms of minerals and vitamins added. Here are some things to keep in mind.

First, check that all minerals are stated in their elemental form. For instance, a product with calcium citrate may read 1000 mg; however, if it doesn't say "elemental," it is most likely that you aren't getting 1000 mg of calcium, but rather a total weight of both the calcium and citrate.

Another common nomenclature practice used by the industry is to place the words Calcium (citrate) 250 mg on the label. This is supposed to indicate that an elemental calcium value of 250 mg is being offered in the form of citrate bound calcium. This might be used, in part, for marketing purposes, since calcium citrate is better absorbed by the body. Other words to look for include ionic, malate, picolinate, aspartate, or the term "Kreb cycle chelates," all of which signify that the manufacturer has formulated its product to enhance the absorption of minerals, ensuring maximum benefit to those taking the supplement.

When it comes to vitamins, make sure you select its natural form. In the case of vitamin E, for example, look on the label for the word d-alpha-tocopherol, which signifies the natural vitamin E, not dl-alpha-tocopherol, which is the synthetic version. (A "d" at the beginning, rather than a "dl," usually connotes "natural.") Natural vitamin E has at least 3 times the biological activity of synthetic vitamin E. Natural vitamin E is a more expensive ingredient and you can be sure of a higher quality product. Some companies have gone really "high-tech" and use co-enzymatic forms of vitamins like pyridoxal-5-phosphate (the active form of vitamin B6) in an attempt to super charge the effectiveness of their products. As in the case of minerals, these forms increase the vitamin's absorption into the body, are more expensive to produce, and usually result in a higher quality product.

A Final Word

Although there are certain high-end vitamin and mineral combinations added to herbal formulas, I want to be clear that a product can still be very effective with less than the very highest form of each ingredient. The goal of choosing herbal formulas with these power-packed forms of nutrients is increased absorption. And you can achieve this when you simply remember to take your non-high-tech formula capsule *without* food, other supplements, or medications—that is, anything that may compete with the product's absorption.

Below you will find listings of herbal formulas I have used successfully over the years. Note that because they are combinations, many contain ingredients not included in this book.

FAVORITE FORMULAS FOR
MEN AND WOMEN

Section I: Herb Combinations for Men

The herbs below have extensive research and/or historical use that demonstrate their benefits to men's health. You will often find several of them combined in formulas:

For General Nutritional, Prostate, and Erectile Support

> Sarsaparilla
> Saw Palmetto
> Ginseng
> Gotu kola
> Licorice*
> Vitamin B6
> Zinc

For Prostate and Erectile Support

> Saw palmetto
> Stinging nettles
> Muira puama
> Zinc

For Erectile Tissue and Prostate Support

> Muira puama
> Beta-sitosterol
> Ginseng
> Gingko
> Saw palmetto

For General Prostate Support

> Saw palmetto
> Pygeum
> Pumpkin Seed Oil

Section II: Herb Combinations for Women

The herbs listed below all have either strong traditional use historically or research supporting their use for women's sexual health and vitality. They, too, are often combined successfully into formulas.

Could be used for PMS, Energy, and Overall Hormonal Support

> Bromelain
> Magnesium
> Vitamin B Complex
> Chaste tree
> Dong quai
> Black cohosh
> Blue cohosh
> Licorice*
> Raspberry

Could be used for Menopausal symptoms, Female Hormone Balancing, and Energy Support

> Black cohosh
> Dong quai
> Licorice*
> St. John's Wort
> Wild Yam
> False Unicorn
> Ginseng
> Sarsaparilla
> Kelp
> Vitamin B Complex
> Vitamin C

Could be used for Formula for Estrogen/Progesterone Balancing

Chaste tree
Saw palmetto
Licorice*
Black cohosh

Could be used for PMS, Hormonal Balancing, Liver Support, and Mild Detoxification

Licorice*
Milk Thistle
Chaste tree
Dong quai
Black cohosh

Could be used for Hormonal Balancing and Detoxification

Wild yam
Chaste tree
Vitamin B6
Dandelion
Black cohosh

*Though licorice is popularly used in numerous formulas, it should be avoided by those individuals suffering from high blood pressure. There is some evidence that licorice increases blood pressure.

Appendix B: RESOURCES FOR FURTHER INFORMATION

I strongly believe that knowledge is power. When I visit with each of my patients, I try to empower them by teaching them about how their bodies work and how the choices they make affect optimal functioning. As questions arise while you read *Better Sex Naturally*, you might choose to contact one or more of the organizations listed in this appendix to gain further information.

It is critical when working with natural medicines to be well informed and have a health care practitioner who can guide you to make the right choices. The naturopathic medical education programs, professional associations, and Web sites included below provide lists of holistic medical doctors and naturopathic physicians around the country and other information that will assist you as you pursue enhanced overall health and sexual vitality. Also provided are a number of resources I routinely recommend to patients, friends, and family who are looking for high quality natural medicine products, and where you can find the herbs discussed in this book.

Naturopathic Medical Education

The following naturopathic medical education programs are accredited (or in candidate status) by the Council on Naturopathic Medical Education, a special body recognized by the United States Department of Education. They are all 4-year, post-graduate programs, and admission requirements are consistent with those of allopathic (M.D.) medical schools. Graduates of these schools are eligible to sit for the examination to be licensed naturopathic doctors (N.D.s). If you are interested in working with an N.D., contact these schools to learn if there are graduates practicing near you.

Canadian College of Naturopathic Medicine
1255 Shepherd Avenue
Toronto, Ontario M4P 1E4
Canada
(416) 498–1255
www.ccnm.edu

Bastyr University
14500 Juanita Drive, NE
Kenmore, Washington 98028
(425) 823–1300
www.bastyr.edu

National College of Naturopathic Medicine
049 Southwest Porter
Portland, Oregon 97201
(503) 499–4343
www.ncnm.edu

Southwest College of Naturopathic Medicine and Health Sciences
2140 East Broadway Road
Tempe, Arizona 85282
(480) 858–9100
www.scnm.edu
(A new naturopathic college was started at Bridgeport University in Connecticut in 1997, but at the time of writing hadn't yet graduated any students.)

Naturopathic Professional Associations

These national associations are comprised of graduates of the above-mentioned naturopathic medical schools. They can also help you find a naturopathic doctor near you, or link you to their state/provincial associations.

American Association of Naturopathic Physicians
601 Valley Street, #105
Seattle, Washington 98109
(206) 298–0126
www.naturopathic.org
(This Web page also has many links to Web sites that offer a wealth of information about natural health care.)

Canadian Naturopathic Association
4174 Dundas Street W, Suite 303
Etobicoke, Ontario M8X 1X3
(416) 233–1043

Holistic Medical Organizations

This group is comprised of active and inactive members. Its members include M.D.s, D.O.s, and N.D.s.

American Holistic Medical Association
4101 Lake Boone Trail, Suite 201
Raleigh, North Carolina 26707
(919) 787–5146

Botanical/Herbal Organizations

These organizations are considered among the nation's leading groups in the field of herbal medicine. They can serve as a resource for gaining additional information on herbal medicine, herbalists, and educational materials.

American Botanical Council
P.O. Box 201660
Austin, Texas 78720
(512) 331–8868
www.herbalgram.org

American Herbalist Guild
P.O. Box 1683
Soquel, California 95073
(831) 475–6219

Herb Research Foundation
1007 Pearl Street
Suite 200
Boulder, Colorado 80302
(303) 449–2265

Useful Web Sites

There must be thousands of natural-health-based Web sites on the Internet. Here are a few that I visit frequently and which I know to have reliable information and/or products.

NaturalMed (www.naturalmed.net)

This Web site offers natural products that meet strict manufacturing standards. I find the site extremely reliable and competitively priced. It also offers free natural treatment protocols for numerous health conditions, and a national list of holistic health care practitioners. The resources it offers includes drug-nutrient interaction listings.

NaturalMedSolutions (www.NatMedSol.com)

This Web site offers the opportunity to review some common approaches to health conditions. It is a great resource.

HealthNotes (www.HealthNotes.com)

Offers information on nutritional and other holistic therapies, along with research citations.

How to Find Quality Herbs

If you've ever stood before a row of vitamin supplements trying to figure out which is best and why one costs twice as much as another, you know that picking herbal supplements to enhance your sex life requires being a knowledgeable consumer. While these supplements are considered food and not regulated or tested by the U.S. Food and Drug Administration, individual manufacturers and suppliers of raw herbs do test and standardize their products and are taking steps to police their industry. They have a long way to go. In 1998, the Los Angeles Times surveyed a variety of supplements available on the market and tested them for the ingredients listed. Some that were supposed to have St. John's Wort had none, while others ranked very well, having more than 90% of what their label stated.

As a shortcut, you may want to contact :

NCNM Natural Health Centers
The Teaching Clinic of the National College of
Naturopathic Medicine
(Natural Medicinary)
11231 SE Market Street
Portland, Oregon 97216
www.ncnm.edu/clinic/medicinary

This is the natural medicine pharmacy of the teaching
clinic of the National College of Naturopathic Medicine,
where I am dean of clinical education. This medicinary
offers more than 2000 high quality products, many of which
are available through its national mail order service.

Below you will also find a list of many companies that
licensed naturopathic doctors trust to provide high-quality
supplements for their patients. These companies provide
products that we stock at the NCNM Health Center. They
work with physicians and herbalists to formulate effective
products, and most of them formulate strictly for profes-
sional-level use; that is, their products can be obtained only
by consulting a physician who is qualified to advise you on
incorporating herbs and vitamins into your health program.
However, some do offer retail over-the-counter products to
consumers and this is noted in parentheses.

Anabolic Labs
17802 Gillette Avenue
Irvine, California 92714

Atrium
10325 North Route 47
Hebron, Illinois 60034

Bezweken
15495 SW Millikan Way
Beaverton, Oregon 97006

BioNativus
(Specializes in high-quality mineral products)
2150 West 3300 South
Ogden, Utah 84401

Biotics Research Corporation
P.O. Box 36888
Houston, Texas 77236

Blessed Herbs
109 Barre Plains Road
Oakham, Massachusetts 01068–9675

Cardiovascular Research
(Serves both the professional and retail market)
1061 B Shavy Circle
Concord, California 94518

DaVinci Laboratories
(Serves both the professional and retail market)
20 New England Drive
Essex Junction, Vermont 05453

Eclectic Institute
(Eclectic has its own herb farm and offers very high-quality herbs to professionals and consumers)
14385 SE Lusted Road
Sandy, Oregon 97055

Gaia Herbs
   (Serves both the professional and retail market)
   108 Island Ford Road
   Brevard, North Carolina 28712–9730

Herb Pharm
   (Serves both the professional and retail market)
   P.O. Box 116
   Williams, Oregon 97544

ITM Herb Products
   2017 SE Hawthorne
   Portland, Oregon 97214

Karuna Corporation
   42 Digital Drive
   Suite 7
   Novato, California 94949

Levine Health Products
   21101 NE 108th Street
   Redmond, Washington 98053–2216

Marz Nutrition
   2002 SE 50th
   Portland, Oregon 97215

Metabolic Maintenance
   P.O. Box 3600
   Sisters, Oregon 97759

Metagenics
   (Serves both the professional and retail market/retail line
called Ethical Nutrients)

1010 Tyinn Street #26
Eugene, Oregon 97402

Nutriwest
11012 Canyon Road East #953
Puyallup, Washington 98373

NF Formulas
(Serves both the professional and retail market)
9775 SW Commerce Circle #C5
Wilsonville, Oregon 97070

Ness
P.O. Box 249
Forsyth, Missouri 66653

Omega Nutrition
(Serves both the professional and retail market)
720 East Washington #103
Sequim, Washington 98382

Oregon's Wild Harvest
(Serves both the professional and retail market)
42464 SE Phelps Road
Sandy, Oregon 97055

Pacific Botanicals
4350 Fish Hatchery Road
Grants Pass, Oregon 97527

Physiologics
6565 Odell Place
Boulder, Colorado 80301

Phytopharmica
    (Serves both the professional and retail market called
Enzymatic Therapies)
    P.O. Box 1745
    Green Bay, WI 54305

Prevail
    (Serves the retail market and has a professional line called
    Tyler Encapsulation)
    2204–8 NW Birdsdale
    Gresham, Oregon 97030

Priority One
    7157 Guide Meridian Road
    Lynden, Washington 98264–9213

Profession Health and Complementary Products
    P.O. Box 80085
    Portland, Oregon 97280

Professional and Technical Service
    (Professional/retail market names: Transitions/Emerita)
    621 SW Alder Suite 900
    Portland, Oregon 97205–3627

Progena
    4820 Eubank Boulevard NE
    Albuquerque, New Mexico 87111

Proper Nutrition
    P.O. Box 13905
    Reading, Pennsylvania 19630

Pure Encapsulations
  490 Boston Post Road
  Sudbury, Massachusetts 01760

Scientific Botanicals
  P.O. Box 31131
  Seattle, Washington 98103

Thorne Research
  P.O. Box 3200
  Sandpoint, Idaho 83864

Trace Mineral Resources
  (They offer a wide array of combination products to the
retail market and specialize in high-quality mineral products)
  1990 West 3300 South
  Ogden, Utah 84401

Western Herbs
  P.O. Box 115
  Index, Washington 98256

Wise Woman Herbals
  P.O. Box 1168
  Creswell, Oregon 97426

Appendix C: GLOSSARY

Acetylcholine:
A chemical neurotransmitter that sends impulses between nerves and muscles.

Adaptogen:
The term given to a plant substance that can help the body by moderating its hormonal response to stress, thereby shielding the body from the physical effects of stress.

Adrenaline:
The lay term for a hormone that is produced and released by the adrenal glands. Its medical term is epinephrine. It also serves to aid and modulate communication between nerves.

Aglycones:
These substances are components of glycosides. They function medicinally as astringents and antioxidants, and also may possess hormonal modulating effects. They include such chemicals as triterpenes, tannins, carotenoids, anthocyanidins, sterols, anthraquinones, etc.

Aldehyde:

A common chemical that has a dramatic effect on the body. For example, acetylaldehyde is a byproduct of the metabolism of alcohol. It is one of the principle substances associated with the feeling of a hangover. When levels become too high, permanent damage or death may result.

Alkaloids:

These naturally occurring plant substances have numerous medicinal properties and are used frequently as drugs (medicinal and non-medicinal). Examples are: yohimbine, ephedrine, caffeine, quinine, nicotine, morphine, atropine, and cocaine. When you see -ine on the end of a chemical name, it is probably an alkaloid.

Androgen:

A category of hormones produced in the adrenal glands, in the testicles, and, to a lesser extent, the ovaries. In men, androgens stimulate male sexual characteristics and functions. In women, androgens modulate several aspects of their well being, including sexual desire.

Antimicrobial:

A substance that can kill or suppress the growth of microorganisms such as bacteria.

Aphrodisiac:

Named for the Greek goddess of love, Aphrodite. Any substance, natural or not, that increases sexual desire.

Atherosclerosis:

The process in which fatty substances and plaques (cellular debris) are deposited in the arteries. As the arteries become clogged with these substances, the body's ability to supply blood is diminished, and with that, the body's ability to receive blood-borne nutrients and oxygen is also diminished.

Ayurveda:

A holistic healing system and philosophy traditionally used by peoples indigenous to India and the surrounding regions, and gaining publicity and popularity in the West.

Benign Prostatic Hyperplasia (BPH):

The disease process that results in the enlargement of the prostate as a result of chemical interactions that trick the prostate into creating additional cells. This enlargement leads to symptoms of urinary frequency and hesitancy, and frequent nighttime urination, and is often accompanied by difficulty achieving erection, diminished libido, and reduced sexual pleasure. As the disease progresses, the entire male reproductive and urinary tract can become affected.

Beta Sitosterol:

A plant substance that has been used to lower cholesterol and is proposed to have the ability to help modulate the effects of sex hormones.

Bioflavonoids:

A term that describes a large category of plant pigments that have medicinal and nutrient properties in the body. The white material on the outside of an orange or grapefruit, for example, is high in bioflavonoids. Bioflavonoids are often also referred to simply as flavonoids, and they increase the absorption of vitamin C (with which they are often found) by up to 35% over the vitamin consumed alone.

Corticosteroids:

Hormones produced by the adrenal glands that function to control fluid and electrolyte balance and nutrient metabolism in the body. They also modulate responsiveness to stress.

Cortisol:

This is a specific corticosteroid that is involved in the fight or flight response. When elevated for a prolonged period of time, however, during extended periods of stress, it lowers immune system function. Cortisol serves as a natural anti-inflammatory agent. This hormone also helps you wake up in the morning by increasing the body's blood sugar levels and revving up your metabolism.

Dehydroepiandrosterone:

DHEA is an adrenal-produced hormone that has gained popularity among health-conscious Americans for its supposed ability to offer a rejuvenating effect for those that consume it. As the human body ages, less DHEA is produced, leading scientists to conjecture that this hormone may be linked to the aging process. Over a period of prolonged stress, DHEA levels can become suppressed, often resulting in premature aging symptoms such as aches and pains.

Dihydrotestosterone:

DHT is a potent form of testosterone that increases as men age. This hormone is associated directly with promoting the swelling and growth of prostate tissue leading to benign prostatic hyperplasia. Herbs and nutrients used to combat BPH act by reducing the production of DHT.

Diverticulitis:

The inflammation and, frequently, the associated infection of sac-like pouches (called diverticuli) in the wall of the colon. This can be an extremely painful condition, and it is thought that stress plays a key role in the development of diverticulitis, along with poor dietary habits.

Double-Blind Study:

A study conducted in a manner that prevents the subjects and the researchers alike from knowing whether the subject is receiving the substance being tested or a placebo (dummy or sugar pill). This form of study is intended to prevent potential bias on the part of researchers (who may be expecting a certain result or outcome), and is the "gold standard" of scientific testing. Sources in the U.S. and British medical communities estimate that 25–35% of all conventional medicine has been tested this way.

Echinacea:

A flowering herb commonly called purple coneflower. It has been called the vitamin C of the herbal world. Echinacea is one of the most popular immunity stimulating herbs in Western Europe and the United States.

Essential Fatty Acids:

These are certain types of fat that must be consumed to maintain health and cannot be manufactured or substituted for by the body. It has been estimated that only 1 out of every 6 Americans consumes sufficient levels of essential fatty acids. They are commonly found in vegetables, nuts, and seeds.

Estrogen:

The primary hormone that produces female characteristics, such as skin tone, hair quality, distribution of weight (breasts and hips), reproductive functioning, and sexual functioning. Men also produce estrogen from special cells in the testes and from the adrenal glands, and it serves numerous functions, including ensuring healthy sperm development.

Extract:

This term refers to concentrated forms of a natural substance. Popular extract types include: solid extracts, tinctures (alcohol or glycerin-based), fluid extracts, and dry powdered extracts. The ratio of an extract refers to its strength in comparison with the raw herb; for example, a 1:2 extract is twice as strong as the herb. The higher the concentration, the more costly the extract will be.

Fibrocystic Breast Disease:

This condition is associated with one or more benign (non-malignant) growths in the breast tissue. This condition is worsened by an imbalance of estrogen and progesterone. Consuming the alkaloid caffeine can also aggravate the condition, increasing the associated pain and the size of the lumps.

Follicle Stimulating Hormone:

FSH is produced in the pituitary gland. Adequate levels are required for the maturation of the eggs and sperm.

Gama Aminobutyric Acid:

GABA is a chemical neurotransmitter that helps dampen and balance the excitatory transmitters and impulses that occur in the brain.

Glycones:

Sugar containing substances frequently found in conjunction with glycosides. They often function medicinally with other plant chemicals to modulate hormonal balance. Common examples include fructose, glucose, xylose, arabinose, rhamnose, etc. Sugars are commonly followed by the letters -ose.

Glycosides:

These are naturally occurring substances that are made up of a sugar component (glycone) and a non-sugar containing component (aglycone).

Homeostasis:

The maintenance of a healthy balance within a specific body system, or within the entire body. Disturbance to homeostasis over time frequently leads to disease.

Hormone:

A hormone is a substance secreted by endocrine glands such as the thyroid, adrenals, ovaries, and testicles. Hormones help control and regulate metabolism and bodily functions. The term endocrinology refers to the study of hormones and their function. An endocrinologist is a medical doctor who specializes in helping patients achieve optimal hormone balance.

Hyperplasia:

The abnormal increase of tissue or an organ resulting from the formation and growth of unneeded new cells. One of the most common occurrences is seen in benign prostatic hyperplasia.

Infusion:
This term applies to the preparation of teas by steeping an herb in preheated water.

Luteinizing Hormone:
Called LH for short, this is a hormone produced by the pituitary gland. It is responsible for regulating egg and sperm production. It also helps regulate production of sex hormones such as estrogen, progesterone, and testosterone.

Lipophilic:
Lipophilic substances are attracted to fatty substances and cell membranes (which contain a fat component), and, as such, possess properties that enable them to pass more effectively into cells and fatty tissue.

Melatonin:
This hormone is produced in the pineal gland, located in the brain. It has gained much popularity as a sleep aid and is taken by travelers to assist them with jet lag. It can affect pituitary hormones, and imbalances cause insomnia and alterations in other hormonal levels in the body that can affect interest in sex.

Nitric Oxide:
A gas that has the ability to dilate blood vessels. Of particular interest is the fact that it increases blood flow to erectile tissue, increasing the firmness and sensitivity of erection in the penis and clitoris.

Palpitation:
An unusually fast or irregular heart beat that is abnormal enough to make a person aware of its occurrence.

Papaverine:
A drug injected into the base of the penis to help men get firmer erections by causing dilation of constricted blood vessels.

Pharmacopeia:
A book that contains a list of drugs or natural medicines and commonly used formulas for health conditions. It may be compiled by either a government agency or by a group practicing a particular kind of medicine, such as homeopathy, and is considered to be an authoritative reference work.

Pheochromocytoma:
A condition in which the adrenal glands produce too much adrenaline and related hormones, which leads to a serious state of overstimulation. This condition warrants continual medical attention.

Phyto-:
A prefix refering to a substance found in plants, such as phytonutrients.

Phytoestrogens:
Substances in plants that function by mimicking estrogen and may be used to regulate estrogen levels in the body.

Phytosterols:
Plant constituents that serve either as precursors to the production of hormones such as progesterone, testosterone, or estrogen, or actually help modulate hormone levels in the body.

Progesterone:

A principal female sex hormone that helps ensure egg maturation and fertility and the maintenance of a pregnancy to completion. It is commonly prescribed to women who have irregularities in their menses, abnormal uterine bleeding, or who may miscarry.

Prolactin:

This hormone occurs in both sexes, though it is most commonly associated with lactation and pregnancy in women. However, elevated prolactin levels can lead to hormonal irregularities in both men and women, such as benign prostatic hyperplasia and premenstrual syndrome, respectively.

Prostaglandins:

These naturally occurring hormones are made throughout the body and are created from essential fatty acids. Some prostaglandins are associated with increased inflammation and lowered immune function, though others are beneficial to the body. Diets low in essential fatty acids or high in fried food and animal products result in imbalances in prostaglandin levels, leading to symptoms such as menstrual cramps, excess menstrual flow, and aches and pains in the body.

Prostate:

This gland sits beneath the bladder and surrounds the male urethra. When the prostate becomes inflamed or swollen, urinary symptoms occur. It is believed that contractions in the prostate during sex add to orgasmic intensity.

Prostatitis:

An inflammation of the prostate. Prostatitis may result from a direct irritant or infection, and may be a consequence of sexually transmitted disease. Symptoms are similar to BPH; see a doctor to find out which is which and what to do.

Pseudoephedrine:

An alkaloid derived from ephedra (Ma Huang). It is commonly used in over-the-counter allergy medicines. At high doses it is a dangerous stimulant, and caution should be exercised even when taking allergy medication as indicated on the label.

Putrefication:

This process arises from an imbalance of protein breakdown that leads to decomposition of food material in the gut. Putrefication most commonly occurs at sufficient levels to cause bodily harm in individuals suffering from constipation, or in those who have an imbalance of "good" and "bad" bacteria in their intestines. Such an imbalance can arise from antibiotic use, exposure to non-friendly bacteria, or insufficient friendly bacteria such as acidophilus and bifido bacterium. This condition can result in hormones that are supposed to be excreted being reabsorbed into the system, creating an imbalance.

Rescue Remedy:

This flower essence product is frequently used by individuals suffering from stress, anxiety, or trepidation.

Saponins:

These are phytochemicals that function to bind certain substances in the intestines, lessening their absorption. For example, saponins are believed to lessen the reabsorption of sex hormones from the intestines, acting to prevent excess levels building up in the blood. Some researchers and clinicians believe saponins also have a direct hormonal effect in the body.

Serotonin:

A neurotransmitter that has numerous functions in the body, most notably its effect on maintaining a level mood. When the body is deficient in serotonin, depression results, and most prescription drugs for depression work by increasing serotonin production. St. John's wort is an example of an herb that has been reported to increase serotonin levels.

St. John's Wort:

A popular herb also known as *Hypericum*. It is used to treat mild depression. It should not be used with other medication taken for depression or anxiety.

Testosterone:

The primary male hormone, responsible for male physical and sexual characteristics such as narrow waist and hips, broad shoulders, muscle mass, and facial hair. It is also the principle hormone responsible for both male and female libido.

Tincture:

These are liquid herbal preparations containing alcohol or a mix of alcohol and water. The end product frequently ranges from 20–50% alcohol, and results in a 1:5 or slightly higher concentration.

Tonic:

The term given to any substance, usually herbal, that provides overall strengthening of one or more systems of the body. Tonics have a moderating effect on body systems, stimulating the fatigued and calming the overstimulated.

Vaginitis:

Inflammation of vaginal tissue. It can arise from infection, over-drying of the tissues (sometimes caused by douching), lack of estrogen to nourish the tissues, imbalance of estrogen and progesterone, or overproduction of cortisol in response to prolonged stress. Atrophic vaginitis occurs relatively frequently in pre-menopausal and menopausal women. It is a common impediment to experiencing enjoyable sex, especially among women during their menopausal years who are either taking nutrients and herbs or hormone replacement therapy.

Wildcrafted:

Wildcrafting refers to the harvesting of herbs and other plants from their native habitat. These plants are considered superior even to organically cultivated herbs because it is thought by some herbalists that the highest medicinal value comes from plants growing in their natural state.

Appendix D: BIBLIOGRAPHY

PDR for Herbal Medicine. NJ: Medical Economics Company, 1998.

Belaiche, P., et al. "Clinical Studies on the Palliative Treatment of Prostatic Adenoma with Extract of Urtica Root." *Phytotherapy Research.* Vol. 5 (1991): 267–9.

Berges, R.R., et al. "Randomized Placebo-Controlled, Double-Blind Clinical Trial of Beta-Sitosterol in Patients with Benign Prostatic Hyperplasia." *Lancet.* Vol. 345 (1995): 1529–32.

Braekman, J. "The Extract of Serenoa Repens in the Treatment of Benign Prostatic Hyperplasia: A Multicenter Open Study." *Current Therapeutic Research.* Vol. 55 (1994): 776–85.

Brinker, F. *Herb Contraindications and Drug Interactions,* 2nd ed. OR: Eclectic Medical Publications, 1998.

Brown, Donald, N.D. *Herbal Prescriptions for Better Health.* CA: Prima Publishing, 1995.

Buck, A.C., et al. "Treatment of Outflow Obstruction Due to Benign Prostatic Hyperplasia with the Pollen Extract, Cernilton: A Double Blind, Placebo Controlled Study." *British Journal of Urology.* Vol. 66, no. 4 (1990): 398–404.

Champlault, G., et al. "A Double-Blind Trial of an Extract of the Plant Serenoa Repens in Benign Prostatic Hyperplasia." *British Journal of Clinical Pharmacology.* Vol. 18 (1984): 461–2.

Chyou, P.H., et al. "A Prospective Study of Alcohol, Diet, and Other Lifestyle Factors in Relation to Obstructive Uropathy." *Prostate.* Vol. 22 (1993): 253–64.

Crellin, John K. and Jane Philpott. *Herbal Medicine Past and Present.* NC: Duke University Press, 1990.

DeRosa, G., et al. "Prolactin Secretion After Beer." *Lancet.* Vol. 2 (1981): 934.

Duke, James A. *The Green Pharmacy*. NY: St. Martin's Paperbacks, 1997.

Dunfour, B., et al. "Trial Controlling the Effects of Pygeum Africanum, Extract on the Functional Symptoms of Prostatic Adenoma." *Annals of Urology*. Vol. 18 (1984): 193–5.

Fahim, W.S., et al. "Effect of Panax Ginseng on Testosterone Levels and Prostate in Male Rats." *Archives of Andrology*. Vol. 8 (1982): 261–3.

Fischer-Rizzi, Susanne. *Medicine of the Earth: Legends, Recipes, Remedies and Cultivation of Healing Plants*. OR: Rudra Press, 1996.

Fouad, Habib K., et al. "Identification of Prostate Inhibitory Substance in a Pollen Extract." *Prostate*. Vol. 26 (1995): 133–139.

Frasseto, G., et al. "Study of the Efficacy and Tolerability of Tandenan 50 in Patients with Prostatic Hypertrophy." *Progresso Medico*. Vol. 42 (1986): 49–52.

Judd, A.M., et al. "Zinc Acutely, Selectively and Reversibly Inhibits Pituitary Prolactin Secretion." *Brain Research*. Vol. 294 (1984): 190–2.

Kappas, A., et al. "Nutrition-Endocrine Interactions: Induction of Reciproal Changes in the Delta-5-Alpha-Reduction of Testosterone and the Cytochrome P-450-Dependent Oxidation of Estradiol by Dietary Macronutrients in Man." *Proceedings of the National Academy of Sciences*. Vol. 80 (1983): 7646–9.

Lahtonen, R. "Zinc and Cadmium Concentrations in Whole Tissues and in Separated Epithelium and Stroma from Human Benign Prostatic Hypertrophic Glands." *Prostate*. Vol. 6 (1985): 177–83.

Landis, Robyn, with Karta Purkh Singh Khalsa. *Herbal Defense: Positioning Yourself to Triumph over Illness and Aging*. NY: Warner Books, Inc., 1997.

Lerner, S.E., et al. "A Review of Erectile Dysfunction: New Insights and More Questions." *Journal of Urology*. Vol. 149 (1993): 1246–55.

Lininger, S., J. Wright, S. Austin, et al. *The Natural Pharmacy*. CA: Prima Publishing, 1998.

Login, I.S., et al. "Zinc May Have a Physiological Role in Regulating Pituitary Prolactin Secretion." *Neuroendocrinology*. Vol. 37 (1983): 317–20.

Mattei, F.M., et al. "Serenoa Repens Extract in the Medical Treatment of Benign Prostatic Hypertrophy." *Urologia*. Vol. 55 (1988): 547–52.

Merz, P.G., et al. "The Effects of a Special Agnus Cactus Extract (BP1095E1) on Prolactin Secretion in Healthy Male Subjects." *Experimental Clinical Endocrinology and Diabetes*. Vol. 104 (1996): 447–53.

Morales, A., et al. "Is Yohimbine Effective in the Treatment of Organic Impotence? Results of a Controlled Trial." *Journal of Urology*. Vol. 137 (1987): 1168–72.

Morely, J.E. "Management of Impotence." *Postgraduate Medicine*. Vol. 93 (1993): 65–72.

Murray, M.T. *Encyclopedia of Nutritional Supplements*. CA: Prima Publishing, 1996.

Murray, M.T. *Healing Power of Herbs*, 2nd ed. CA: Prima Publishing, 1995.

Murray, M.T. and J. Pizzorno. *Encyclopedia of Natural Medicine*, 2nd ed. CA: Prima Publishing, 1998.

Ody, Penelope. *The Complete Medicinal Herbal.* NY: Dorling Kindersley, 1993.

Reid, Daniel. *A Handbook of Chinese Healing Herbs.* MA: Shambhala Publications, 1995.

Romics, I. "Observations with Bazoton in the Management of Prostatic Hyperplasia." *International Urology and Nephrology.* Vol. 19 (1987): 293–7.

Scott, W.W. "The Lipids of the Prostatic Fluid, Seminal Fluid and Enlarged Prostate Gland in Man." *Journal of Urology.* Vol. 41 (1939): 406–11.

Shibata, O., et al. "Chemistry and Pharmacology of Panax." *Economic and Medicinal Plant Research.* Vol. 1 (1985): 217–84.

Sikora, R., et al. "Gingko Biloba Extract in the Therapy of Erectile Dysfunction." *Journal of Urology.* Vol. 141 (1989): 188A.

Simonsen, U., et al. "Nitric Oxide Is Involved in the Inhibitory Neurotransmission and Endothelium-Dependent Relation of Human Small Penile Arteries." *Clinical Science.* Vol. 92, No. 3 (1997): 269- 75.

Sinquin, G., et al. "Testosterone Metabolism by Homogenates of Human Prostates with Benign Hyperplastic Effects of Zinc, Cadmium, and Other Bivalent Cations." *Journal of Steroid Biochemistry.* Vol. 20 (1984): 733–80.

Sohn, M., et al. "Gingko Biloba Extract in the Therapy of Erectile Dysfunction." *Journal of Sex Education and Therapy.* Vol. 17 (1991): 53–61.

Susset, J.G., et al. "Effect of Yohimbine Hydrochloride on Erectile Impotence: A Double-Blind Study." *Journal of Urology.* Vol. 141 (1989): 1360–3.

Teeguarden, R. *Radiant Health.* NY: Warner Books Inc., 1998.

Wagner, H., et al. "Search for the Antiprostatic Principle of Stinging Nettle (Urtica Dioica) Roots." *Phytomedicine.* Vol. 1 (1994): 213–24.

Waynberg, J. "Aphrodisiacs: Contribution of the Clinical Validation of the Traditional Use of Ptychopetalum Guyanna." Paper presented at The First International Congress on Ethnopharmacology, Strasbourg, France, June 5–9, 1990.

Weiss, R.F. *Herbal Medicine.* Stuttgart, Germany: Hippokrates Verlag, 1985.

Werbach, M.R. and M.T. Murray. *Botanical Influences on Illness.* CA: Third Line Press, 1994.

Werbach, M.R. *Nutritional Influences on Illness*, 2nd ed. CA: Third Line Press, 1996.

Werbach, M.R. *Foundation of Nutritional Medicine*. CA: Third Line Press, 1997.

White, J.R., et al. "Enhanced Sexual Behavior in Exercising Men." *Archives of Sexual Behavior*. Vol. 19 (1990): 193–209.

Wren, R.C. *Potter's New Cyclopaedia of Botanical Drugs and Preparations*. Cambridge, U.K.: C.W. Daniel Company Limited, 1988.

Zaichick, V.Y., et al. "Zinc Concentration in Human Prostatic Fluid: Normal, Chronic Prostatitis, Adenoma and Cancer." *International Urology and Nephrology*. Vol. 28 (1996): 687–94.

INDEX